RAINBOW RELATIVES

Real-World Stories and Advice on How to Talk to Kids About LGBTQ+ Families and Friends

SUDI "RICK" KARATAS

Skyhorse Publishing

This book is dedicated to nieces and nephews Jamie,
Jo Jo, Tony, Brian, Kara, and Danny.

Skyhorse Publishing books may be purchased in bulk at special discounts
for sales promotion, corporate gifts, fund-raising, or educational purposes.
Special editions can also be created to specifications. For details, contact
the Special Sales Department, Skyhorse Publishing, 307 West 36th Street,
11th Floor, New York, NY 10018 or info@skyhorsepublishing.com.

Skyhorse® and Skyhorse Publishing® are registered trademarks of Skyhorse
Publishing, Inc.®, a Delaware corporation.

Visit our website at www.skyhorsepublishing.com.

10 9 8 7 6 5 4 3 2

Library of Congress Cataloging-in-Publication Data is available on file.

Cover design by Jane Sheppard

Print ISBN: 978-1-5107-3173-8
Ebook ISBN: 978-1-5107-3174-5

Printed in the United States of America

Contents

Introduction

The idea for this book was born during a phone conversation with my sister, who lives with her family in another state. I had asked if her three school-aged kids knew about my sexual orientation. She said she wasn't sure and wondered how and when to tell them. She paused for a moment and then said, "I wish there was a book on that." That night, I decided I should write that book.

Not only did I not know if my nieces and nephews were aware that I was gay, but I wasn't even sure if some of my adult relatives knew. Many of them live outside the United States and I don't see them often enough that the topic had ever come up. It had been hard enough when I finally decided to tell my parents and brothers and sisters—I had waited until I was in my thirties. Even today, in an age when it's supposed to be much easier and more accepted, I know many gay adults in their thirties and forties who are still not out to their parents. Will it ever become easier for families to have this conversation?

I decided the best way to find out was to talk to others who have been in my shoes about how they handled it. How did their families react? How did the children in their families react? I collected stories from friends, acquaintances, and strangers. I sent out surveys and interviewed people who are LGBTQ (Lesbian, Gay, Bisexual, Transgender, Queer). I talked with straight people who have gay relatives. I asked every demographic of LGBTQ parents and even children of LGBTQ parents about their experiences. I also interviewed some therapists and some openly gay/lesbian/transgender celebrities. Many of the names used in the stories and surveys have been changed, except where people gave permission to use their real names.

This book is not based on science or textbook theories, just real stories from real people. It's intended to be a straightforward, informative, entertaining, and humorous guide to help parents, uncles, aunts, teachers, and other trusted adults find the language and methods to discuss and educate children (ages three to seventeen) on the subject of nontraditional sexuality. It considers families from all different cultural and religious backgrounds and is especially geared toward helping those who live in more conservative communities. A number of books deal with the topic of "coming out," but very few focus on the kids who are related to, or are simply close to, the people who come out.

This is the first book to tackle this topic directly and to demonstrate different ways that real individuals have explained the diversity of sexuality to kids. Even more important, as I learned from many people I interviewed, this book will also help us learn from kids and their mostly accepting and unpretentious reactions. Perhaps the most important thing that I learned from writing this book, and through the many great films, books, and people that I was exposed to, is that kids are much more aware than they get credit for, and this is a conversation every one of them should have, whether or not it relates to a family member.

You may find the stories educational and entertaining, even if certain subjects don't apply to you specifically. Some testimonials may simply help you feel like you are not alone and provide you with some comfort. If you are seeking some quick tips in certain areas, these can be found in boxes that contain approved materials from several organizations like PFLAG, Family Equality Council, and COLAGE, among others.

Each chapter has stories, interviews, or experiences that either offer advice or allow you to draw your own conclusions to decide what is best for your family. I add my own two cents here and there as well. As such, you'll notice that some of the advice and opinions may vary or even contradict each other. An approach to having these conversations with your children is not set in stone nor one size fits all; every child is different, as is every situation, so please take what you need from what you read and feel free to toss the rest. These are just ideas to inspire families to have these conversations.

We'll begin with a chapter about LGBTQ aunts, uncles, and family members. This opening chapter is very dear to my heart, as it reflects my experiences as a gay uncle. We'll then move into speaking with children about parents who come out as LGBTQ and then consider the children's perspectives as we discuss what they may encounter in places they frequent, such as school and church. Psychologists, therapists, and a few celebrities will weigh in with advice they've drawn from their own experiences with clients or family and friends, and then we'll wrap up with some information on communities, peer groups, and media that may help you talk to your children about—and help your children understand—their LGBTQ family members.

I hope you enjoy *Rainbow Relatives* and find it helpful for your families.

—Sudi (aka Rick) Karatas

CHAPTER 1

A Monster Wasn't In Your Closet (But Your Uncle Was)

When my nephew was thirteen years old, his Christmas wish list included the movie *I Now Pronounce You Chuck and Larry*, a movie about two men pretending to be gay and getting married for health-care benefits. He was already an Adam Sandler fan and thought the premise of the movie sounded pretty funny. At the time, I wondered if he might be too young for a movie with that subject matter and thought perhaps it was better if he didn't see it. (Okay, so maybe I thought he shouldn't see it because it had a ridiculous plot.) But I was also concerned because I had no idea if my nephew knew his uncle is what Chuck and Larry were pretending to be. I decided not to buy it for him, but someone else bought him the movie anyway.

Is Younger Better?

As I did research for this book, I realized not only was my nephew old enough to watch a film with a gay theme, but that

1

younger is probably better for children to be introduced to people who are different in a few ways yet the same in so many others. The consensus of the people I interviewed was that it's easier to be more accepting at an earlier age before kids are exposed to outside influences that may lead to forming negative beliefs or homophobia.

I'm not saying it's a good idea to throw in *Brokeback Mountain* or *Queer as Folk* between episodes of *Sesame Street*, but by the time kids get to elementary school, they should not equate gay people with aliens from outer space. The more they know, the less of a big deal it seems—and it really isn't a big deal at all. The more it's kept a secret and not talked about, the more taboo, wrong, and shameful it may seem and the bigger the issue becomes.

Many gay people I spoke to were like me in that they simply weren't sure if their nieces or nephews knew. Many people don't live near their families, or they don't have a boyfriend or girlfriend around enough in their daily lives, so the kids didn't have the chance to put it together on their own. However, in some families, the subject just wasn't tackled or talked about. Period.

To Tell or Not to Tell, That Is the Question

Every family and situation is different. Questions that often arise include: Who gets to decide when a child should know? What if the parents don't want their kids to know about their aunt or uncle yet, but the aunt or uncle wants their nieces and nephews to know? Should the aunt or uncle have to hide who they are or pretend that they're someone other than themselves? What if they have a significant other whom they would like to bring to family gatherings just like everyone else?

One person I interviewed at the Los Angeles Gay Pride Parade put it simply: "When children see two people in a loving relationship, it's not really talked about. They just see that this couple love[s] each other, and as they get older they just understand. They are not told unless they ask. So it's more of a coming to know. They just see a relative with someone else in a relationship of the same gender, and they kind of just get it."

I interviewed one person who had a nephew who was nine years old. He said to his uncle, "I hope you find someone to love like Aunt Barbara has." Aunt Barbara had a female lover. The kid figured it out by himself. He had never been told his uncle was gay, but somehow he knew.

Discussions

Avoiding the discussion of gay issues with children can end up harming everyone involved. Silence isn't going to change someone's sexual orientation or make it go away; it only makes it seem wrong or shameful. It's a matter of not just letting kids know about LGBTQ relatives, but also making sure their questions and concerns continue to be addressed. It's likely that children will hear some classmates make negative comments about LGBTQ people, or they'll see prejudice on TV or social media. They may see news coverage of many states trying to pass anti-LGBTQ laws, like those allowing someone to deny service to an LGBTQ person if it's against their religious beliefs. In fact, in February of 2014, Arizona did pass a law of this nature, but the governor later vetoed it.

A lot has changed even in the past few years I've spent writing this book. While it's certainly becoming easier to be out or openly gay in today's world, conflicting messages are still being put out there as debates over gay rights continue to ignite sala-cious talk in the media.

Questions and Answers on Coming Out to Nieces and Nephews

Much of the research for this book came from surveys I asked a number of people to fill out. In many of them, on the subject of when and how to tell children about their relatives' sexual orientation, the adults indicated they were nervous about how the kids would react, while most of the kids indicated that the news didn't bother them at all. The following are some of the questions and answers taken from the surveys to give you a feel for the basis of my research.

Do your nieces and nephews know you are gay? If yes, how old were they when they were told or found out? How were they told? How did they react? If they have not been told, why not?

- **Paul:** Yes. They were about nine and eleven when they found out. My niece was the one who "outed" the situa-tion, so to speak. My sister and I had been on the phone and I was talking about my boyfriend. When she got off the phone, her daughter said, "Who were you talking to?" She said, "It's your uncle." Her daughter laughed and said, "No, you were talking about someone and their boyfriend." That opened up the dialogue for my sister to explain to her daughter that her uncle was gay. She listened and took everything in stride. She wasn't offended or freaked out. But the funniest part was at the end of the conversation when she said, "I only have one question . . . does that mean I have lesbian blood in me?" My sister laughed a little and was more shocked that her daughter even knew the term *lesbian*. She then informed her daughter that her uncle being gay has nothing to do with her [own] sexuality. My niece said, "Cool . . . and no wonder he dresses so well." Ha! Later that day she explained it to my nephew. They had to be a little more gentle with him because he looks so much like me and so many people tell him that; they wanted to make sure that [he understood] people wouldn't "assume" he was gay because of the similarities. Luckily, he was fine with it too. Neither has ever shown me any resentment or bias. Impressive, since they live in Middle America.

- **Sandra:** [My kids] found out when they were ten and twelve years old. My son realized there was only one bed in the apartment my brother shared [with his boyfriend] and came right out and asked if he was gay. I said yes—I knew that they probably already knew.

- **Eddie:** I never "came out" and said "I'm gay," but I never hid it from [my nieces and nephews]; they all met my partner and figured it out. I don't censor my speech or my actions around them. If I did, it would imply there's something wrong with it.

- **Rosa:** Yes, at age nine, my niece saw a picture of me and my partner and asked her mom, my sister, if I was gay. My sister replied yes. A bit later my sister asked her if she had any questions—and she said no.

What were some questions they asked, and how were they answered? Did boys react differently than girls? How?

- **Allen:** They asked, "Do they love each other?" And things like "What's a lesbian?" or "What's a gay person?" My response was, "They are with a person of the same sex, just like people are with people of the opposite sex, and there's nothing wrong with that!"
- **Adrienne:** They didn't ask questions—I asked them an important question. "Now that you know that your uncle is gay—do you feel any differently about him?" Their immediate response was no.
- **Trevor:** The girls were more vocal about not caring. The boys were quieter.
- **Alastair:** When my nephew found out, he said he didn't want to talk about it.
- **Sybil:** The girls wanted to know the love story; [the] boys didn't ask, just accepted without questions.

Do you have any other comments or suggestions?

- **Michael:** Don't underestimate the understanding and unconditional love of a child—especially in this day and age. Everyone knows someone who is gay; it's no big deal anymore.
- **Ellen:** I don't discuss my sister's relationship with her husband to my children and did not feel the need to discuss my brother's relationship [with his partner] either. Their sexual preference does not define them and my children should not (and don't) treat them any different now that they know.

- **Tig:** Kids are very smart and are aware of many things. Don't ever dodge the sexuality issue and your kids will grow up to be more respectful and well-rounded.
- **Mia:** Be yourself in front of family. When they ask, answer them honestly and at their maturity level. They all were happy when I married my partner of thirty years.

How old do you think children should be when they are told?

- **Pat:** [You should tell them] as early as possible. The older they get, the more they have to overcome. [My nephew] never batted an eye at us cuddled on the couch.
- **Annie:** I'm going to wait until they get older . . . junior or high school. Younger than that, I feel they won't be mature enough to understand. But they know I have a special, healthy, and happy relationship with a person they see me with all the time, so by the time I tell them, they might already anticipate and understand it's perfectly normal to have that type of relationship.
- **Albert:** Children should always be raised with a vocabulary that's inclusive of gay culture.
- **Raul:** Nowadays, they learn everything by age four or five.
- **Sam:** It depends on the maturity level of the children.
- **Inga:** I think that once they understand dating and sexual relationships, it's an appropriate time to tell them. My niece and nephew clearly understood the difference between homosexual and heterosexual and weren't as offended or shocked as we thought they would be. With the characters on TV and film, it's not foreign to them anymore.

Do you have any advice on speaking with children on this subject?

- **Ambrose:** Since heterosexuals don't go out of their way to discuss sex with their nephews and nieces, I don't see any reason for gay uncles to either. It is probably best to answer if asked. The closest we got to a discussion was when discussing politics. I said that, as a gay man, it would be difficult to vote Republican.
- **Nancy:** Don't make a big deal of it. Present it as a normal way of life. Don't use alternative language. It just is.
- **Cory:** [When to tell them] depends upon the child—let them ask when they are ready. If a gay couple simply lives their lives as a couple, it will be a natural occurrence for the child.
- **Bart:** I think kids today are a lot smarter and more aware than we give them credit for. They understand that a person can be just like Mom and Dad but like, and love, someone of the same sex. And that it's okay.
- **Isobel:** It only becomes a big deal if you make it a big deal. Treat it like a normal, everyday thing (which is how it should be treated) and kids won't care. If you act strangely, they will pick up on it and think being gay or lesbian is strange.
- **Will:** Talk to them like adults (without graphic details). They probably won't care as much as many adults. Don't act nervous or as if you are about to tell them something bad.
- **Ursula:** I think just being a positive example speaks for itself.

The Pink Elephant In the Room

In my interview with Tommy Woelful and Richard Vaughn, I asked their thoughts on how and when nieces and nephews should be told. Tommy said that when they visited his family in Texas, their relationship had always been "The Great Big Pink Elephant in the Room." (It was the first time I've heard this expression and I couldn't help but love it.) When his sisters' kids were finally told at a family reunion, one of his nephews, who was about twelve years old at the time, said to Richard jokingly, "What do we call you, Auntie Rich?"

Tommy's sister quickly jumped in, defending her brother-in-law. "You call him uncle. There are many different types of people and families and you need to respect them all," she told her son.

The lesson here was clearly not to make fun of others because they are different and to always show respect, and I'm sure it had an impact.

Real Stories: How Kids Found Out

The Cell Phone Kiss

The following is a true and touching story told to me by a good friend. The names here—and in most of these stories—have been changed.

Hank's thirteen-year-old son happened to pick up a cell phone that his uncle (we'll call him Bert) had left in a room. The boy began looking at the pictures saved on the phone. He came upon one of his uncle Bert locking lips with another man (we'll call him Ernie). The boy didn't say anything to his dad, who knew his brother was gay, but he did mention it to his mom. She casually mentioned the incident to Hank.

When Hank was in the car alone with his son, he brought up the subject. He said, "I heard you saw a picture of Uncle Bert and another man kissing."

"Uh, yeah," said the boy, uncomfortably.

Hank said, "You mean like on the cheek?"

"No," said the boy, squirming.

Hank continued, "On the lips?"

"Yes," replied his son, awkwardly.

The father said, "What are you saying? My brother is gay?"

"I don't know!" the boy blurted out, embarrassed and fully believing that he was the one breaking the news to his father.

Hank let his son squirm for a while and then finally let him off the hook, telling him he already knew and it was fine and not a big deal at all. Then Hank made his son promise not to tell his younger brother yet. They would when he was older and ready.

They say a picture is worth a thousand words. If you don't want kids in your family to know yet, and there is any chance you might risk leaving your cell phone lying around where they might get their hands on it, then you better make darn sure there are no incriminating pictures on it or remember to lock it with a pattern or code! And if you have Grindr on your cell, that could be your undoing as well.

Hank decided to wait to tell his youngest child, which he felt was right, and it was completely his right to make that decision. However, quite a few people I spoke to suggested that it's usually better to tell all the children at once so that none of them are put in the position of harboring secrets or spilling the beans in a less than appropriate way for their younger sibling to digest.

Regina's Robe Inquiry

Back in the 1970s, when Regina was about five or six years old, she had asked her mom, "Why does Uncle Ben wear a girl's robe?" The robe she was referring to was made of silk and decorated with bright flowers, and it hung way above his knees and almost up to his butt (as Regina put it).

Her mom said, "Well, Uncle Ben is a model," which he was, "and they like to dress differently sometimes and like pretty clothes." Of course, not all gay men wear feminine clothes like flowery short robes, but some happen to, and that is what made Regina ask a question. Her mother didn't tell her that her uncle was gay (which was probably harder to do in the 1970s), but she did tell Roberta that he liked to dress a certain way.

When Regina was a few years older, she would always see her uncle Ben with the same gorgeous guy (we'll call him Jerry). That was when Regina's mom told her that her uncle was gay and that Ben and Jerry loved each other. Regina remembers that she had been completely fine with all this and didn't think it was a big deal at all. In fact, she remembers saying to her mom, "Oh, okay, can I have some ice cream?" And they went to Baskin-Robbins.

Marti's Modern Parenting

My friend Marti is originally from New York and now resides in the San Francisco Bay Area in California. She allowed me to include a few of her own experiences speaking with her son, Billy, when he was younger, about her gay cousin.

Once, at Marti's cousin's house—Mark and Chuck had been together for nearly twenty years—she took Billy to the bathroom and he asked, "Mama? Those guys, Mark and Chuck . . . They're brothers?"

"No," she replied, "not brothers."

"Hm," he said. "Is there a mommy who lives here?"

"No," she said, "just Uncle Mark and Uncle Chuck."

"Oh," he says, nodding happily. "I get it! They're like two dads!" A proud moment for Marti. Simple. Simple. Simple. "That's right," she said, "just like that." Billy was almost four years old at the time.

Another time, Billy said, "Mama, boys and girls dance together like this," and he proceeded to do a toddler's best attempt at a waltz with an imaginary partner.

So Marti said, "That's true, Billy, boys and girls do dance together like that . . . and sometimes boys dance like that with boys, and girls dance like that with girls too."

And he said, "You're right, Mama. I think Uncle Mark and Uncle Chuck dance like that too! Don't you think so, Mama?" He understood that love is dancing together cheek to cheek.

Mr. Wilson's Neighborhood

Mr. Wilson says he knows his nieces and nephews know he's gay, but he's not sure how they know or how they were told. It's not something that has ever been talked about, but he's been in a relationship for over forty-five years with the same man, so it is really just understood. A good, long relationship speaks for itself.

Mr. Wilson once had an eight-year-old neighbor (we'll call him Dennis) who asked, "Are you gay?" Apparently, another neighbor had told him he should stay away from Mr. Wilson because he was gay.

Mr. Wilson told him yes, he was gay.

Then Dennis asked, "What does gay mean?"

Mr. Wilson replied, "You should talk to your parents." Two months later, Dennis and his family moved. Was it a coincidence? Who knows?

Adolfo's Anxieties about Coming Out to His Nephew

Adolfo, who lives in Florida, told me that his nephew didn't know that his uncle is attracted to *hombres* (the Spanish word for men). When the boy was about eight years old, he went to dinner with his uncle Adolfo and his male "friend." The "friend" took some food from Adolfo's plate and ate it. The nephew said, "That is weird. Only married people should take food from someone's plate." Kids are *very* observant!

When his nephew was twelve, Adolfo went to dinner with his sister, his mom, and a few other friends, including a new couple who didn't know about Adolfo's orientation. The subject of relationships came up. The nephew asked, "Why doesn't Uncle Adolfo have a girlfriend?" Adolfo didn't necessarily want this new couple to know he was gay, but at the same time, he wanted to answer his nephew's question.

Then someone else added to the pressure, "Yes, you're very good looking. Why don't you have a girlfriend?" Adolfo did not feel comfortable answering the question that night.

Finally, six months later, Adolfo decided to come out to his nephew, who at that point was almost thirteen years old. Adolfo's sister had left him to decide when he wanted to share this with her son. He decided to do it on their way to the airport to pick up the boy's grandmother because he'd have an hour in the car with him to talk it through. Adolfo was nervous; he had planned to have the conversation a few times already, but had always backed out. He always had a good time with his nephew and didn't want that relationship to change. He was scared of being rejected by his nephew. He finally said, "I have something very personal I want to talk to you about. I haven't spoken about it before because I always felt you were too little, but you really will always be too little to me. Even when you are forty years old, you will still be too little."

Before he could talk himself out of it, he said to his nephew, "You are very important to me. I know you wonder why I am not married and why I don't have a girlfriend and you are worried that I am alone. I want you to know I am not alone. I do have somebody, a special someone. Let me ask you something, do you understand what *gay* means?"

The nephew said, "When a man loves another man." Then the nephew added, "There are two gay kids at school and they're very nice."

Adolfo said, "That is what I am trying to tell you. I am gay." Adolfo became emotional but tried to remain calm and collected as he asked his nephew if he had suspected. His nephew replied that he actually had no idea and was shocked. He had not connected any of the dots. Adolfo asked if he had any questions.

His nephew said, "I have so many thoughts in my head."

Adolfo said to him, "I want an honest relationship with you. This is the only thing I was hiding from you, the only thing you didn't know about me. You are probably going to have questions and I want you to come to me with any of them."

The nephew said, "I just want you to be happy."

Adolfo said, "You know the person I am with. Do you want to guess who it is?"

The nephew said a little uncomfortably, "I don't know, I don't know." Adolfo told him who it was. The nephew had met him several times at family events.

When they got to the airport, they got something to eat and drink like they always did: a tuna sandwich and a soda. They had always shared the same straw but after their conversation, Adolfo thought the nephew might ask for a different straw. He didn't; he seemed fine. His nephew asked if Grandma knew. Adolfo said everyone knew, including Grandma, who probably took it the hardest because she was "old school" from Peru. His nephew laughed at this. Adolfo made sure his nephew knew that nothing had changed between them. When he got back home that day, he'd lain down for an afternoon nap and slept a very, very peaceful three hours. He'd felt as though something very heavy had been lifted off his shoulders. Hiding something does require a tremendous amount of energy.

About a week after coming out to his nephew, they were watching *The Amazing Race* on TV and someone said Adolfo should go on that show. His nephew then said, "Uncle Adolfo would do very well on *The Amazing Race* because he is smart and strong." Adolfo's being gay did not affect his nephew or their relationship in any way.

"You Dress Like a Boy."

Jo is gender nonconforming. Gender nonconformity is behaving and appearing in ways that are considered atypical for one's gender. When she spoke to me, she had a five-year-old nephew whom she has been very close to since he was a baby and who still likes to spend a lot of time with his aunt Jo. One day, the boy looked closely at his aunt Jo and had a sudden realization.

He said to her, "You dress like a boy and wear your hair like a boy. Why?"

Jo answered, "It's the way I like to dress and wear my hair. We all should look the way we want to and wear what we like and do what makes us happy. Like the way you sometimes prefer to wear shorts." He was very content with this answer. Sometime later, Jo's sister had been giving away some of her clothes as well as some of her husband's clothes, and the boy didn't question why Aunt Jo would be more interested in his dad's clothes and not his mom's based on the previous conversation.

Jo's nephew goes to a progressive school where LGBTQ subjects are openly discussed and some of the students have even said they feel they may be transgender, even at that early age. Jo told me that when her nephew's parents were telling him about gay marriage and how his aunt Jo would be getting married to a woman, all the nephew cared about was, "When do I give the rings?" He was extremely excited about the whole wedding and the part he was playing in it and couldn't care less who his aunt was marrying.

Lesson from Liza (No, Not Minnelli)

One woman I spoke to told me about the experience she had with her family in the early 1990s. Liza was in her twenties when she came out, and her niece was three years old at the time. The little girl had approached an adult visiting their home one day and announced, "My auntie Liza has a wife."

The adult replied, "Well, my brother John has a husband."

To that, the little girl simply responded, "Oh, okay."

I've seen Liza's experience reflected in the majority of surveys and interviews I conducted with people who have come out at different times throughout the decades: someone being gay is no big deal to a child, especially a younger child with minimal social biases to affect their opinions. When someone comes out later or the child is told when they're older, it seems that more "loss" is incurred, including loss of expectations.

One of the things I learned from my interviews and surveys is that parents make the mistake of thinking that if they have to tell their kids about gay people, then they have to talk about sex. They don't.

For example, John Dennem, who I interviewed for chapter 8, told me his nephew was told John was gay when he was about five years old. He has always been fine with it, asking simple questions such as whether or not Uncle Johnny and "so and so" slept in the same bed. They were mostly innocent questions based on the logistics of there being only one bed in the spare bedroom and the kid's innocent concern over where his uncle would sleep when he came to visit with his partner. In fact, most questions he asked were about comprehending, in a child's mind, how things would work with two men in one bed. The inquiries were not about sex but comfort.

Throughout my research, many people suggested explaining sexual orientation in an age-appropriate context for their kids. Parents can explain that their uncle, who happens to spend most of his time with the same guy or an aunt who spends most of her time with the same woman, do so because they love each other, the same way Mommy and Daddy do. Keep it as simple as that. Most children don't seem to have many issues with this, and if it were a perfect world, that would be the end of it. But we don't live in a perfect world, do we?

CHAPTER 2

Daddy Left Mommy for Tommy
(When a Parent Comes Out as Gay)

I like to view things with a sense of humor (hence the title of this chapter). However, it can be a serious family matter when one parent comes out as LGBTQ. The situation will often result in a divorce, which can be devastating for a child and can result in their conflicting feelings of anger, sadness, confusion, and self-blame.

During the early 1980s, when I was in high school, I remember watching a movie alone with the volume turned low because it was such a controversial subject for that time. The film was called *Making Love*, and it came out (pardon the pun) in 1982, starring Michael Ontkean, Harry Hamlin, and Kate Jackson. Ontkean plays Zach, who is married to Claire (Jackson). Zach is gone so much that Claire believes he is having an affair with another woman. When she confronts him, he admits his affair with his patient, Bart (Hamlin). Back then, many believed that playing a gay role hurt Hamlin's career for years, whereas today such roles have actually bolstered many careers. In 2005, *Brokeback Mountain* won a number of awards and was nominated for best picture at the Oscars. In 2009, Sean Penn won the best actor Oscar for his performance of controversial gay rights activist Harvey Milk. In 2014, Jared Leto won the Oscar for best supporting actor for his compelling role as a transgender woman in the film *Dallas Buyers Club*.

However, while these movies certainly helped to bring the LGBTQ community into popular culture, they did not portray situations that directly involve kids. In 2011, *The Kids Are All Right* became one of the first movies to do so with its portrayal of a lesbian couple raising two children born from a surrogate father. The film won a Golden Globe for best picture and was nominated for an Independent Spirit Award for best screenplay. Hopefully, this has opened the door for more film and television portrayals depicting the reality of children with LGBTQ parents and the common situations that result when one parent turns out to be gay.

When a Parent Comes Out

The following is an amusing story told to me by a friend: A man was married many years to a woman and together they had a daughter. When the daughter was almost grown, the man came out to his family, announcing he was gay. He wasn't sure how the daughter was handling it until one day, as they were both taking a walk along the beach, two very attractive and muscular men were walking toward them, each carrying a surfboard. His daughter said, "Look, Dad, one for you, one for me."

The father was relieved, seeing how comfortable his daughter was with his sexuality. So he joked, "Okay, I'll take the blond."

Embarrassed and turning red, the daughter said, "I was talking about the surfboards."

I spoke with and surveyed a number of other people who had been married and had children when one spouse came out. Hopefully, some of the following stories will help those who are in similar situations, and they will be comforted to know they are not alone.

Honesty is the Best Policy

After fifteen years of marriage, Anna and her husband sat down together with the kids and told them about her husband's sexual orientation. The kids were fourteen, twelve, and eight years old. They were sad and surprised, but they were relieved to know there was a valid reason as to why their parents had separated. Prior to that, no one could understand why this had happened because they'd always had a good relationship together.

"My advice to others going through this is to be honest with everyone involved and tell people as soon as you are comfortable," Anna said. "If you do it too soon, you may wind up hurting yourself and the people around you, especially the children. My kids did not want anyone else to know because they studied in the same schools as their cousins. I couldn't tell any of our relatives because children can be cruel at school. I would have liked to tell people sooner but my kids would have been hurt."

Hide That Gay Porn

After a year of being separated from his wife of twenty years, Fred's sons were visiting him from Texas. At that time, they were thirteen and fifteen years old. He had told his wife he was

gay, though he'd never acted on it, and they had decided to separate. However, they had decided not to tell the kids the reason
until it came up during his sons' visit.

While his sons were visiting, his fifteen-year-old left the
room to take a shower when his thirteen-year-old asked him,
"Are you gay?" Taken aback, Fred asked, "Why do you ask?" His
son said, "Well, you used to watch both straight porn and gay
porn on the internet and now you only watch gay porn."

The fact that his thirteen-year-old knew how to find the
porn that he thought he had hidden so well was a little scary.
(Kids today are very computer savvy, if you haven't noticed.)

"My son was actually okay with it," Fred said. "I told my other
son a couple weeks later and he laughed at first—he thought it
was a big joke. Once he knew it wasn't, he was okay with it, too,
until they got back to Texas and their religious school. Then
they told me I was an embarrassment because everyone gave
them a hard time about it. Today they are both adults and fine
with it."

An Author's Advice

I interviewed Rick Foster, who cowrote a book with his partner,
Greg Hicks, and Jen Seda, MD called *Choosing Brilliant Health*. I
had met him during a seminar they did at an Actors Fund work-
shop. Rick had been married with children when he came out in
the 1980s, but since they lived in San Francisco, it was a little easier to do than in, for example, a small town in upstate New York
or somewhere in Mississippi, Alabama, or Texas. He had already
moved out when he told his fourteen-year-old daughter, but he said
that many of the fears about coming out to her were never actual-
ized. He told her, "You know Greg, my best friend? He and I have

a sexual relationship. We're a couple. I need you to know I do not have AIDS. I am HIV negative. I am not putting on a dress. I am the same person. I just have sex with Greg." (Keep in mind, this was back in the late 1980s, when many more people were dying from AIDS and it was a much bigger concern to the public.)

She asked, "Why are you telling me now and not Alex?" referring to her brother, who was three years younger.

He said, "Because you are older."

She asked, "Who else knows?"

He gave her a list of people who knew and told her, "If you need support, they are there for you."

Then she caught him off guard and said, "How do you know I haven't had sex with women?" It was a clever way of turning the tables to get her father to react, but she had only been teasing him.

About eight months later, Rick wanted to bring his boyfriend, Greg, to see one of his daughter's performances at the school. She allowed it, but told her father, "Don't talk to anyone at the school or let teachers know you are gay because you'll embarrass me." She meant that she didn't want him making a big deal out of his sexual orientation because so many of her friends had gay parents. If he made a special case out of it, then it would be embarrassing. During her senior year, as a proud daughter, she gave a speech about having a gay dad.

Rick's experience with his daughter reinforced his belief that "it's very important to stay involved in your kids' lives." His story clearly shows that coming out to your children isn't just a one-time effort and then it's over. Kids have different phases at different ages and may go back and forth with their feelings. Parents need to be present and understanding throughout all of it and realize that sometimes it may take time.

Rick decided to come out sooner to his son. He waited until the boy was eleven and they were faced with a six-hour drive from San Francisco to LA. Rick said, "There's something I need to discuss with you. Greg and I are in a gay relationship, we have sex, no impact on your life."

His son's response was common for the time: he'd asked, "Do you have AIDS?" Rick said that once he finally told his son he was gay, it was like the floodgates opened. His son opened up to him about many things for the first time and also asked if it would be okay if he told his friends. Rick told him it was okay as long as he was comfortable doing so.

Rick offered some suggestions for others to keep in mind when telling the kids in their lives:

- Don't treat it like a trauma.
- Make the kids the top priority.
- Have other loving adults in their lives in place as a support group. Tell certain friends who know the kids well, and tell teachers that you can trust to be understanding.
- It is also important to evaluate the children's community environment. For example, consider whether or not there are negative stigmas in the community or if you live in a homophobic or violent neighborhood and determine how to handle it.

Dealing with a Bitter Spouse

Sometimes when one parent comes out, their spouse resents it and causes a rift or even sabotages the relationship between the gay parent and child. This may make it difficult for the child to understand and accept their gay parent, but it doesn't make it impossible. Take Waylon's experience, for example.

Waylon was divorced, and his ex-wife did not take his being gay very well at all. Waylon's daughter lived with his ex-wife and her new husband while Waylon provided financial support for his daughter but lived in another state. The relationship was strained for a long time because of the negative things his ex-wife would say about him and his sexual orientation. The daughter also didn't know that other family members had accepted her father for who he was. When Waylon's daughter was sixteen, she finally visited her dad and his partner, Willie. Not surprisingly, it was a little awkward at first, but he assured her that their relationship wouldn't change. He asked her if she'd get to know Willie, since he was important to him.

She asked questions about their relationship—how long they'd been together, how the relationship was going in general—and she also had her own private conversation with Willie and asked him questions as well. She was able to see that her father's relationship with Willie was no different from other relationships, and by the end of the day, she had even given Willie a hug.

However, once she returned home to her mom and stepdad, the situation became more difficult. Waylon soon got a call from his furious ex-wife, Maybelle. "How dare you introduce my daughter to this lifestyle!" She continued to flood him with homophobic voice mails, emails, and even threats. Maybelle never did come around; in fact, she tried to poison her daughter against her ex-husband with lies about him and used parental alienation to prevent her daughter from seeing her father.

The daughter was finally told the truth, and the relationship between Waylon and his daughter (who recently came out as gay herself) is now healthy and strong.

I think it's good that Waylon showed his daughter that he and Willie have a nice, loving relationship that offset the negative things his ex had said. Setting a good example is important. I think when one spouse (in this case, the mother) has resentment toward a divorced spouse, it causes a lot of harm to a child, and if any adult finds themselves pitting the child against the other parent in situations like these, they should, of course, do their best to stop.

When the Kids Don't Take the News So Well

Pablo's son was ten and his daughter was seven when he came out to them. Pablo had decided to tell them because he thought his ex-wife was about to out him. He later told his kids that he needed to tell them because he didn't want them to find out from a third person. He started by saying to them, "I've got something important to tell you." But then he couldn't continue.

The three of them sat in awkward silence until his son finally said, "What are you going to tell us? That you're gay?" Pablo was surprised but relieved. "Yes, that's why your mom and I separated." He then told them, "I am still your father, nothing changes, and I still love you the same way."

Then, both kids started crying. The boy seemed to take it harder than his sister, throwing a puzzle across the room in apparent anger. The crying lasted about fifteen minutes or so, and then later the son suddenly said to him, "Daddy, I'm sorry for those comments and jokes I've said about fags before. Don't take them personally, but I am still going to make them." It was the boy's way of trying to use a little humor to break the tension. Pablo said this didn't bother him too much because if his son felt free enough to make a joke at this time, he felt his son was partly okay with it. Pablo said he also understood the "macho thing" boys have and his reaction was fairly normal.

His son asked, "Did you ever love Mommy?"

He said, "Of course." But although the conversation seemed to have resolved things at the time, Pablo told me that his kids didn't believe that he was born gay for quite a while, and today his son is still not 100 percent okay with it, but their relationship is okay. The daughter is much better with it.

I think the takeaway here is even if you fear the kids won't be okay with this news, it's still better to be open and honest and give them time to adjust to it.

Advice from Amie Shea on When and How to Tell the Children

I interviewed Amie Shea, one of the founders of the Gay Dad Project. Her father came out as gay and divorced her mother when she was a teenager. Amie offers some very helpful advice for kids and parents who are faced with this situation. She says that the sooner parents can tell the kids, the better, to ensure there is a good support system in place. The situation can cause resentment and be extremely emotional for the kids and the ex-spouse. She advises kids not to ignore their feelings, including anger, confusion, and fear. In fact, she says it's okay to be mad, but it's also important to think about the reasons for feeling such anger. She also tells kids there are plenty of people out there for them to talk to. "Parents are afraid the kids may reject them, and that is why they don't come out for a long time, so kids should try to understand that," Amie explains. However, she also reminds parents, "The hardest thing is that there can be trust issues for some. The parents lied about this; what else did they lie about?"

I watched a video on the Gay Dad Project website and found it to be an extremely interesting sample of the documentary to come. It is a clip from an interview with a gay father who tells his story about when he came out to his wife and them both having to tell their kids they would be getting a divorce. He said, "I told my wife, let's just tell the kids we're getting divorced, let's just tell them we can't get along and then later on we'll deal with the rest. Divorce is gonna be hard enough for them, let's not do it all at once." His wife did not agree and told him, "No, you're wrong, the most important thing now is the truth and it's not easy, but we have to tell them the truth and we have to do it now." I'd argue she was right.

Cody and His Very Accepting Son

I saw Cody Renegar, in the documentary film *Hollywood To Dollywood*, and I was so moved by what he said in it that I contacted him for an interview. He had been married to a woman, and together they had a son, Levi, who is now in his late teens. In the film, Cody tells a great story about when he came out to his son. Levi was barely four years old at the time and had already been hearing plenty of derogatory comments about his father being gay. The little boy had been riding with him in the car when he suddenly piped up from the back seat, "Daddy, what does *gay* mean?"

Cody said, "It means I'll let a man love me the way Mommy loved me."

His son thought for a moment, then said, "I don't care who loves you, as long as someone loves you."

When Levi was eight, Cody asked him, "Would you rather that your father had been straight?"

Levi answered, "That would be weird!"

However, little Levi grew up and there was a period during his years in junior high school that he didn't want his dad and his dad's boyfriend attending the school football games or functions. Some of the kids had been calling Levi a fag. Cody only found this out later because his son didn't want to hurt his feelings by telling him.

During Levi's time at his conservative school in Arkansas, Cody and his partner had also tried to place an announcement of their engagement in the local paper, which wouldn't allow a same-sex marriage announcement. Cody and his fiancé fought for their right and posted their plight online. It went viral and ended up on the local news. Cody was worried about the type of attention his son would receive in response to the news story, so he met with the teachers on how to handle the situation. They were very supportive and would pull Levi out of class just to ask how he was doing. The teachers also made sure to tell Levi that his dads were heroes. Other people in the community also began recognizing them for their bravery.

Whenever Levi would tell his dad that someone had said something negative about gay people, Cody would ask him, "Did you help them understand?" Cody also suggested that his son invite more friends over to the house to help them realize they were just like any other family. It worked.

I asked Cody if there were any benefits to raising kids as a gay parent. He gave an interesting response. "It is good to have something different or unique about your childhood that helps you see the world as it really is, and see the beauty in it, even in the face of adversity. I try to make sure who I am doesn't affect my son in a negative way. It is important to show your child that you're human with flaws but that you are trying to overcome them. It's good for them to see a parent becoming stronger against the odds. I tell my son, let the kids know that if other kids tease about anything, it is their problem, not [his]."

Years later, Levi shared his own perspective of his father in an interview, saying, "After all the things my dad has been through in his life, I can't believe he is still nice."

Cody, who I now call a friend, is one of the nicest guys you could ever meet and has a great sense of humor. More importantly, he has proven to be a great parent with great values, which will surely be passed on to Levi.

Tips for Coming Out to Your Kids from COLAGE

- **It's never too early to come out to your children.** Kids understand love; what they don't understand is deception or hiding. And it's never too late to come out to your child. COLAGE has met folks in their forties whose parents are just now coming out to them. Often knowing the truth will be a relief for kids of all ages.
- **Tell your children in a private space where the conversation can't be overheard and will be completely confidential.** Telling them at your regular Saturday night dinner at your favorite restaurant could be overwhelming.

(continued)

- **Make sure you tell them when there will be plenty of time for the conversation to continue if it needs to.** For example, if they are staying with you for the weekend, talk with the kids on Saturday morning instead of waiting until the drive back to their other home on Sunday night.
- **Try writing it down first or practicing with a friend if you're nervous.**
- **Their reactions are going to vary.** Some may need some time and space to process the information on their own. Some might have a million questions. Others may barely react at all. No matter how your kids respond to your coming out, honor the process that they need to go through for themselves.
- **Listen and ask your children what they already know and feel about LGBTQ people.** Both as a starting point to have a discussion about sexual orientation, as well as in regard to suspicions they may have had about you.
- **Don't think that coming out to your kids means it's time to have "the big sex talk."** Explain your sexuality in age-appropriate ways and in ways that they can understand. Talk about having feelings of love, care, and concern, along with attraction, for the same sex. If you are involved with someone and feel comfortable sharing this information, it's a good idea [to do so] as you will be explaining your feelings for someone your kids know. Being able to discuss a relationship with another person

can make the whole thing more grounded and less abstract.

- **Think of this as a lifelong conversation, not a one-time deal.** Your children's thoughts, feelings, and questions will continue over time and will change as they get older. This month they might not care, next month they might be mortified, next year they may have lots of questions. Keep the conversation alive; the tricky part is avoiding them feeling like you want to talk about it *all* the time (but believe me, that's better than not enough).

- **Let them know that you love them no matter what.** One of the main things kids worry about is that you will no longer share the common interests that you used to, or that you will somehow be different than you used to be. At the time of coming out, some parents do go through what we fondly refer to as a "second adolescence." Let your kids know that you are happy and are enjoying a new aspect of your life, but that no matter what, they are your number-one priority. And then prove it to them by being consistent, attentive, and communicative.

- **Help break down stereotypes of LGBTQ people for them.** If your children already know other LGBTQ people, draw comparisons between you and them. If they don't, tell them things that may seem obvious to you, like not all gay men are hairdressers; give examples of famous LGBTQ people whom they

(continued)

can look up to. They may be concerned that your whole personality is going to change now that they know you are gay, lesbian, bisexual, transgender, etc.; reassure them that you are still you—being LGBTQ is simply one more thing about you. There is no one way that all LGBTQ people must act.

- **Give them options of other supportive adults to talk with.** Sometimes it's easier for kids to express some of their feelings with another adult because they don't want to hurt your feelings. If one of your parents, siblings, or friends is being especially supportive or there is another adult that you trust, arrange for them to spend time with the kids to provide a sounding board.

- **Your kids may be gay. They may be straight.** Either way, it's not a judgment on your parenting. Nor are they doomed to a life of loneliness and desperation and homophobia (if they are gay). Be as supportive of your kid's orientation as you wish your parents were of yours.

- **Respect your kids' wishes about how, when, and who they come out to about you.** Let them tell their friends, peers, and others at their own pace and in their own time. Recognize that now they, too, have the joy and burden of coming out.

- **Most importantly, connect them with other kids who have LGBTQ parents.** Studies show that when children know they are not alone and have opportunities to share with other kids with LGBTQ parents, they have fewer problems. Go to events with your local LGBTQ family group if there is one; go to Family Week, cosponsored by COLAGE and Family Equality Council, in the summer; buy books for them about gay families; have the kids join online groups run by COLAGE; become COLAGE members so your family can connect to other families in your area. Just let them know they are part of a community that cares and understands. They are not alone. Millions of other kids have experienced what they are now going through and there are ways that they can connect to this caring community of peers.

Advice and Insight from Kids of LGBTQ Parents from COLAGE Literature

- "My advice to parents is to come out *clearly*—and not just once, but several times in different ways. There should be the 'sit down at home and have a frank talk about it' version. (And remember: coming out as a LGBTQ person doesn't have to include talk about sex.) Then there should be reminder/check-in discussions, as in 'What did you think of that gay character in the movie?' or 'What do you want to do for Gay Pride month?' or 'How do you feel about putting this rainbow sticker on the family car?' Just as your coming-out process was probably gradual, your

(continued)

kid(s)' process will take place over a period of time. Being honest from the beginning will save a lot of grief later." —Meema, New York City, New York

- "I often hear that children are smart and can pick up on a lot. A few years before my dad came out to me, I suspected that it was true. Unfortunately, before my dad told me, I had already found a card from a man he had been dating. My advice to parents in the process of coming out to their kids is, the sooner the better. In your coming-out process, be as open and honest as you can. Make the situation a positive thing in your child's life. Be confident in your decisions and know that your child loves you for you, and not your sexuality." —Amber, Lawrence, Kansas

- "When my mum came out to me more than four years ago, I wasn't upset about it. The idea of having two mums was very exciting and I felt, and still feel, like it was a huge bonus for me. To me it feels like there can't be anything better than having two mums. I was never upset that my mum was a lesbian, only worried about the difficulties that it would entail. Though I came across some problems at school, I feel that my family situation has made me a stronger and better person. It really makes you appreciate everything that you have. I'd never change my mums' sexuality. It's a blessing." —Hannah, United Kingdom

- "Tell your kids as soon as possible—it's better that they hear it from you than from anyone else. Also,

if you have more than one child, try and tell them
all at the same time. Otherwise you will put the
kids that know in a difficult situation of not telling
their siblings. When this happened to me, although
I was okay with the idea of having a gay parent, I
was uncomfortable with it being a secret. Being
as open and honest as possible about your sexual
orientation will model to your kids that difference is
not something for which you need to be ashamed."
—Max, San Francisco, California

- "When my mom came out to me, she just slipped
it into a casual conversation. It felt uncomfortable,
awkward, and a total surprise. I wish that my mom
would have said something like, 'I have something
that I want to talk to you about. It might sound
surprising and I'm not sure how you will take it.
I've had some realizations about my feelings in
relationships. I am starting a relationship with
a woman and I feel very much in love with her.
What do you think about what I just said?'" —Lisa,
Portland, Oregon

- "When I was in third grade, my mom went to her
friend Debbie's wedding. When I asked her how it
went, she told me she had a lot of fun dancing with
Kathy . . . I laughed and said 'Duh, Mom, what are
you, gay?' She said, 'Actually I am.' This is the first
time I really understood what she meant by 'I love
Kathy' (her partner). Don't ask her about it, though . . .

(continued)

she swears that's not how it happened." —Diane, Kingston, Rhode Island

- "My advice is don't sweep it under the rug or assume that it doesn't affect your children because it is simply *your* identity. In fact, it changes the dynamic of your entire family and the way in which they'll see themselves in relationship to other families. Your children will likely be very sensitive to the homophobic images and comments they are exposed to. It's not always easy for children to understand, especially when they have not yet formed their own identities. Never hide your relationships. If your children are raised around honest and loving relationships, they will be more likely to enter the world with a strong sense of the legitimacy of their family and personal identity. By being a visible LGBTQ parental presence, you can help affirm the normalcy of your existence for you, your children, and the society in which they will raise their children."
—Ava, Wellesley, Massachusetts

What the Therapist Says: Divorce + Gay Parent = Added Shame

As part of my research, I also spoke with therapist David Giella. I reveal more of our interview in chapter 8, but he provided some very straightforward insight into what children of gay parents go through in these situations. "In any divorce where, let's say, the father has an affair, the child may feel the following: 'You misled Mommy; you made Mommy cry; you had an affair; you have screwed up my life because of something you did; I'm scared and mad at you.' When the father has an affair with another man, it's mostly the same feelings, except now the child has to deal with having a parent who is gay, and there may be some shame with this, whether there should be or not," Giella said.

I think what Dr. Giella said is important because parents should be aware a divorce may be a little harder for kids to deal with when it's because one parent is gay. It's an additional change and something else to adjust to in their lives; it's not as simple as their parents not being together anymore.

That Certain Summer

In my research, I came across an old treasure trove of a film called *That Certain Summer*, which was shown in 1972 and was way ahead of its time. Hal Holbrook plays Doug, a man who gets a divorce because he is gay. His son doesn't know why his parents split up until he visits his dad and meets his dad's much-younger "best friend," played by Martin Sheen (who seems extremely comfortable with his masculinity, as he can be seen on the show *Grace and Frankie* on Netflix, again playing a gay man).

Doug's ex-wife is played by Hope Lange, who learns to accept her ex-husband's new lifestyle and convinces him to tell their son. It was the first TV movie to tackle the subject of homosexuality but was very tame compared to what is on television today. I was eight when this movie came out, before I realized I was gay. However, I do wish there had been more films like it during my youth.

I think my friend Frank Velasquez summed it up nicely for parents who may be afraid of coming out to their kids or being rejected. "I learned that my kids love me unconditionally. If you know deep in your heart that they love you, as you love them, everything will work out just fine."

CHAPTER 3

Two Moms, Two Dads, Today's Families

Many of the families in the previous chapter were already formed when a parent came out and usually it was a surprise to the kids and many adjustments had to be made. Now we will hear from some same-sex couples who decide to adopt or have children through a surrogate or in vitro fertilization. Being a parent and raising a family is not easy. Is it harder if you don't have a traditional family? Since I don't have kids, I relied on the interviews and surveys to get a better understanding of the challenges these families face. I will leave most of the advice to them and let their answers speak for themselves.

LGBTQ Parents
If you could give advice to other gay/lesbian/bisexual/transgender parents or same-sex couples with kids or thinking of having them, what would it be?

- **Andrew:** I think that it's the most amazing thing I've done . . . and the hardest. I've learned more about myself in this journey (both good and bad). Someone gave us the advice that if Oliver ever says, "I want a mommy," to think about it as if he said, "I want a horse." Our son doesn't know what a mommy does versus his daddies . . . and it will keep us from feeling like we're depriving him of something.
- **Thea:** It's awesome, but only do it if you are 100 percent sure. I always thought I wanted a biological child but I could not love my adopted kids more.
- **Bruce:** Having kids, it's the greatest thing ever.
- **Primrose:** Adopt from foster care! So many kids in our own cities and states need parents.
- **Albert:** Make sure you are both on the same page; it makes life better when you both know what the other is thinking.
- **Kathy:** Join an organization such as Pop Luck Club (PLC), an organization in Los Angeles, California, made up of families with two dads and go to Maybe Baby (a fertility group). Seek out other gay parents. Visit with other families, be a camp counselor, go read to kids in schools, volunteer. If you have never been in charge of other kids, like mentioned above, then it can be tough; already knowing how kids act can really help.
- **Ted:** Do it. It's the best gift in the world.

Were there any issues, challenges, or interesting stories (serious, humorous, or heartwarming) at school or other social settings regarding your kids having a gay/lesbian/bisexual/transgender parent?

- **Andrew:** On Mother's Day we were going to brunch, two dads and our son, and a woman stopped us on the street and said, "It was nice to give mom the morning off." We pointed out that Oliver didn't have a mother but that he had two dads and she said, "I'm going to pray for you and remember Jesus loves you," and she then crossed the street. I thought the woman's reaction was rude, while my partner thought she was being nice. I don't know what her motivation was for saying it, so I decided to be happy someone was praying for us.

- **Daniel:** One main issue that continued to come up in their early years was other parents' confusion when our children stated that they had two dads. Classmates usually didn't care, but they did mention their parents said that our lifestyle was "wrong."

- **Eduardo:** We've really encountered very few negative responses when people learn we are gay parents. I expect this will get a little more complicated as they move out of the private preschool into public school. We try to prepare them gradually for the reality of how some people think badly of gay people and gay parents. For example, I recently donated some money to help some gay Ugandans escape Uganda. We talked about that and how there are some places in the world where people like their dads might be hurt or killed for loving each other.

- **Frank:** I am a stay-at-home dad in a very "soccer mom" area. Going to the grocery store always brings on comments, and of course the old Southern ladies ask the most questions. When they say, "Your wife must love that you do the shopping and take your daughter," I smile and say, "My husband lets me be a Real Househusband of Atlanta." Their looks are priceless.

- **George:** Tough time was at Mother's Day when the boys would make something for a grandmother or aunt. I would talk to teachers ahead of time, but they usually forgot. Most classmates didn't care. Having worked with kids before and being very present at their schools helps offset any weirdness. When applying to schools, I always asked if there were any other same-sex parents at the school.

- **Harry:** It's liberal here, so not too big an issue; I don't think it even came up at all in preschool. In kindergarten, an older kid came up to me and asked, "Does Wes really have two dads?" I said, "Yeah," and he said, "Oh," and went about his playing. They have told him he *must* have a mother somewhere, a birth mother at least, and he's asked about his birth mother and we tell him again how a woman grew him in her tummy for us. It's a bit confusing since her name is the same as about three of our friends!

- **Igor:** He has a classmate (with two gay dads) who came out of the same tummy as his sister (!) and that hasn't been an issue. It's probably actually helped, because it makes gay dads less unusual and he's not the only one. I really do think *Will & Grace*, *Modern Family*, and Facebook have helped the country accept gays.

- **Julie:** My churchy conservative friends from school days see me and my family on Facebook and I think it must give them pause at first. I wonder, are they going to reject us because we're gay? But they haven't and now they get to see we're pretty normal folk, with granite-cleaning issues and stain-removal questions. We don't have after-hours parties and thongs. I have family members who stopped watching *Friends* because of the gay wedding, and now *Modern Family* is their favorite show, so we've come a long way pretty quickly.

- **Ted:** Not yet. We did put a I LOVE MY DADS T-shirt on the boys and the teachers at school "love the shirts." I heard that about two or three times when I went to pick up the boys, who are two and five years old.

What are some questions your kids have asked about having a gay/lesbian/transgender parent? How old were they when

they asked, and how did you answer? Describe the coming-out process.

- **Julie:** We have a nineteen-year-old daughter and a twenty-one-year-old son. Some of the questions they asked at ten and thirteen years old were things like, "How are we supposed to respond to people saying that our lifestyle is wrong? How are we supposed to make friends?" Our first response to their question was that they cannot always change the way people view others. Also, that true friends would judge them on their friendship, not their parents' sexuality. We never actually came out to them—we were out before the children came into our lives.

- **Kelsey:** We have a six-year-old boy and an almost three-year-old girl. Our son sometimes is into bridal dresses, and asked if we got married and when. We told him we had, then he asked, "Which one of you wore a bridal gown?"

  I said, "Neither of us. We're both men, so we both wore regular clothes. We got married during a heat wave and the ceremony was outside, so we just wore regular clothes." (I realize now that we could have worn dresses!)

  Then our son asked, "If two women get married, how do they decide which one wears a gown?"

  "They both could, or neither could—it's up to them; it's their wedding, so they can do what they want."

He was probably four years old at the time. We didn't have to come out since they've been with us since birth and they know and see other gay and single parents, so they know there are all sorts of families. When school starts, it is clear most families have a mom and a dad, so it comes up. He has been around pregnant women, and he knew they were carrying babies, so we have told him, "We really, really, really wanted a baby, and since we're two men and babies only grow in women's tummies, a woman grew you in her tummy for us."

What do you feel are some of the benefits of raising kids as an LGBTQ parent? What are some benefits for the children?

- **Katie:** The ability to show them, firsthand, about love and diversity. And the ability to teach them about and exercise tolerance.
- **Lauren:** The obvious advantage is that most gay parents have their kids on purpose. (Almost) no accidental pregnancies in our group! I think gay parents tend to be very accepting of their kids being different from our expectations for them. We know what it's like not to be accepted by our parents and we try very hard to love our own kids unconditionally.
- **Lawrence:** We have loving homes, with two parents that really wanted children, who have to not only put a lot of time but money into having a family.

- **Michelle:** LGBT parents can be more open to recognizing depression, bullying, or even just holding back. I think it promotes a healthy attitude towards sexuality and being able to talk to your kids about sex when the time comes. Hopefully, it'll help kids learn to be more understanding of others.
- **Maurice:** We have a lot of friends who don't have children, so our daughter is very lucky to have so many people love her.
- **Ted:** I'd like to think we have a built-in "accept everyone" policy in the household. And I think it's easier to say, "be whomever you want to be."

What are some of the disadvantages of having LGBTQ parents?

- **Nico:** People expressing their opinions can be very cruel.
- **Nannette:** Our kids are likely to be exposed to discrimination and negativity about their families, but it can be character-building as long as it isn't too extreme.
- **Oliver:** People asking about their mom or why I'm not married . . . I don't want my kids to feel different. I want them to feel loved!
- **Paul:** Possibility for being picked on, and, if single, you definitely need a strong female presence from an aunt, grandma, or friend.
- **Ted:** Well, life as we know it. They will get ugliness. And we'll be here to remind them there is more happy than ugly in the world.

Many of the topics, issues, and inspiring comments that came up in the surveys were common among the families. To get more of a feel of households with same-sex parents, I did a few personal interviews and have shared them with you in the following pages.

Some Modern Family Stories

A Progressive Family in the Conservative South

Tommy Starling is on the board of the Family Equality Council and lives in South Carolina with his husband, Jeff Littlefield. Together they're raising two children. At the time I interviewed Tommy for this book, their daughter, Carrigan, was seven years old and they had a newborn son named Braxton. Aware that South Carolina is a very conservative place, Tommy was only half joking when he told me they might be the only openly gay couple in the entire state. But Tommy also makes a strong point: "The way to change people's attitudes and minds is to get involved in the school and the community, so the parents and neighbors get to know you and see how you really are."

When they first brought their daughter to school, they were met with some resistance from other parents. Then Tommy decided to run for the school board. Threatened by his candidacy, somebody sent an anonymous, nasty letter out to the community and basically told everyone not to vote for him. After all, he was gay and that meant he had no moral values and would teach their children bad things. The school was also reluctant to have him run. So Tommy sent an email to the board chair inviting everyone to a poolside event, where he would serve ice tea and lemonade, welcoming anyone who wished to come meet him. He also promised to answer any questions or concerns about what his morals and beliefs were and to explain what he intended to do to help the school and community. The invitation was enough to indicate how open and sincere he was. The board decided the gathering wasn't necessary, and not only did the school allow him to run, but he won by a landslide with 85 percent of the vote.

You don't have to win an election to win people over, but Tommy really emphasizes that the key to being accepted by a community is to be a strong part of it. "By being very involved, and getting out there and letting them get to see who you are, and how much you care about your kids, is what changes their attitudes," he explains. "This way, you build a huge support system, and have allies with many straight families to offset or knock down negative attitudes in the community of those who were against them." He also says, "Being parents trumps being gay. If they see you are a good parent, that's all that matters."

We also discussed religion. Tommy and Jeff were both raised in very religious families. A lot of preachers came out of Tommy's family, and Jeff was raised as a Mormon. Neither one of them stayed with their religions after they both felt burned by their churches. However, they still allow their daughter to go to church with her friends, where she enjoys learning the songs. When she comes home and reports that she learned things like "God created everything," they simply ask her, "How do you know that?" Their goal in asking such questions is to make her think for herself, rather than encouraging her to believe everything she is told. They also teach her that everyone has different beliefs, and will allow her to choose what to believe when she gets older, but she must always treat everyone with respect, regardless of their beliefs.

Tommy and Jeff have also helped their daughter come up with ways to handle things at school. A classmate had asked her, "Where is your mom?" Carrigan simply replied that she didn't have a mom. The other girl pressed on: "You have to have a mom and dad!" Carrigan said, "Nope, I have two dads." As Carrigan stood her ground, the discussion actually got a little heated and the teacher (who had been coached on how to handle this situation as well) stepped in. "There are a lot of types of families and we need to have respect for all," the teacher told Carrigan's classmate.

Tommy also allowed me to share one of his Facebook posts from March 2014:

> *There is hope for the South! Tonight, while picking Carrigan up from dance class, one of her seven-year-old friends came up to me and the following conversation occurred:*
>
> **Seven-year-old**: *Does Carrigan really have two dads?*
> **Me**: *Yes.*
> **Seven-year-old**: *Why?*
> **Me**: *Because that is the way we decided to make our family.*
> **Seven-year-old**: *So she has two dads . . . what about a mom?*
> **Me**: *She doesn't have a mom, she just has her two dads.*
> **Seven-year-old:** *Well, that is not fair!*
> **Me**: *It's not? Why?*
> **Seven-year-old:** *Because . . . I want two dads. Dads are really cool. But my mom is a good cook. Which one of you cooks?*
> **Me**: *We both cook, but I cook the most.*

Seven-year-old: *Well, that's cool. Here comes Carrigan. See you Thursday.*

Lesson: *Children do not know to judge or discriminate unless they are taught to do so. They understand more than people think. Simple answers to simple questions are all they need. And to the parents of this child, thank you. —Her two dads.*

Tommy shared another encouraging post on Facebook in February 2018:

> We often focus on the negative things that happen to us, so I wanted to point out something that really touched my heart recently. A couple of parents, teachers, and friends from our children's school came up to us to thank us for being in this community and opening their children's eyes to diversity. A couple of the comments were "My kids are more open-minded and accepting because of you guys" and "Because you guys are here, my kids don't blink an eye to seeing or hearing about two-dad or two-mom families. They never would have been exposed to that without you." It's really nice to know we make a difference to many people and that there are some who actually appreciate us. It's even nicer to hear it from time to time.

Soccer Dads

I interviewed a wonderful couple, Richard Vaughn and Tommy Woelfel, who lived in Southern California with their five-year-old twin boys, Aidan and Austin. I had the opportunity to watch their sons tear up the field in a soccer game and then spent some time interviewing Richard and Tommy for the book.

Richard is the founding partner at the International Fertility Law Group, whose mission is providing individuals and their families with the highest caliber legal support in all aspects of assisted reproductive technology law, including surrogacy, egg donation, embryo donation, sperm donation, parental rights, nontraditional family formation, co-parenting, and second-parent adoption. Tommy is a certified indoor cycling instructor and actor. Together, they have created a beautiful family unit, and it was really cool to see them enjoying their sons' soccer game as two dads. A couple of their friends also came to give their support as well. Ten or fifteen years ago, two dads at a soccer game would have certainly raised eyebrows—and in some places, I'm sure it still does—but hopefully this is becoming a more normal thing and will eventually be accepted even in the most conservative communities.

Until then, Richard and Tommy have been very aware of where they bring the children up. They had considered moving to one of LA's beach communities because of the good schools, but decided against it because, due to the lack of diversity, the communities remain very conservative. They felt the kids would have a better experience where they are now.

They have also found a great church. The Beverly Hills All Saints Episcopal Church is a progressive church that has a gay pastor and female ministers as well. Most of the students and parents at the school also don't have any issues with their family. Neither do the neighbors.

Richard and Tommy were married while it was legal in California, just before their boys were born. Then Prop 8 passed and suddenly same-sex marriage was illegal in California. The twins were about three and a half when Tommy and Rich tried to explain the situation to them. The kids only knew that if you do something illegal, you could get a ticket. So they asked, "Are you getting a ticket?" When Prop 8 was overturned and gay marriage was again legal, the boys were happy to know that no one would be getting tickets.

When asked what they see as some of the advantages of a kid having two dads, they said one advantage is that many kids have absent fathers while their kids have two dads who are each paternal and maternal.

Bullying, Adoption, and Having a Support Network

John Ireland is the board president of the Pop Luck Club, a great support group that celebrates gay dads. He has two children, Giovanni and Emma. When I spoke with John, he mentioned that a relative had asked him, "Why would you parent a child when you know they will be teased and called names?"

He replied, "Kids are bullied for everything. Children are teased for being adopted. The kids will say in a negative way, 'You're adopted,' even if they weren't implying there is something wrong with that. Kind of like the expression 'You're so gay.' It is said in a negative way. Kids will make mean comments no matter what."

When his kids come home upset about something another child has said to them, or something they've overheard, he tells them: "Whenever someone says something negative about gay people or if they have a problem with our family, just feel bad for them. They probably don't have a lot of friends." At the same time, he also told them, "No one has a right to talk about our families. Nothing about us, without us." He has realized the importance of kids speaking from their own experience to affirm and defend themselves. Children need to be taught to be resilient and encouraged to overcome adversity, regardless of whether they're adopted.

John talked more on the subject of adoption: "As far as adoption goes, it is not an LGBT right; it is a matter of suitable parents. What is in the best interest of the child? Will they have a safe and loving home? Is that being denied to the child?"

According to John, a popular concern some people have for a child with two dads or two moms is that the child misses out on having a mother or a father, respectively. To illustrate this point, he told me about his uncle-like relationship with the four-year-old daughter of a lesbian couple he is good friends with. One day he had been sitting in their living room with the girl, who was resting on his chest. Suddenly, she said, "I love you, Daddy." This upset her two mothers. Kids do notice a missing mother or father. Because of this, John said, "It's important to have a support network of people; it takes a village. For example, if you are two dads, perhaps you should develop a strong group of women for your kids to know. Make sure the kids have women in their lives that function in a maternal, caring way. Find people who will support them and provide them with safety and nurturing."

Raising Kids in A Two-Dad Family

When I interviewed Stuart Bell, who authored the book *Prayer Warriors* (under his pre-married name Stuart Howell Miller), he talked about raising kids in a two-dad family. His son was fortunate in that he went to a private school, where there were actually quite a few other children who had two moms or two dads. He said, "Parents can't protect their children from the world. All you can do as parents is create as much support as you can. Other kids or people are going to make fun no matter what. Someone is too fat, too poor, wears glasses. Kids are made stronger and they learn to deal with the real world." Stuart added, "It's also just as important to work out your own issues as a parent."

During our conversation, we discussed whether he felt a child needs a mother. Stuart said, "I have never really felt that a child needs a mother. I do feel that society places a huge emphasis on children having a mother and I have had concerns about how society's views would hurt my child." Stuart came to the conclusion that what a child needs is love and support. Stuart made a very important point, saying, "The biggest concern in having children is their safety and happiness, so if you deal with those issues [regarding missing parental figures in the home], that is what is important."

Although there are some challenges to raising a child as a pair of gay parents—Sometimes we do come across some homophobia, like when we were visiting back in my hometown in Tennessee. We had our eight-month-old son at a restaurant and someone overheard a waiter say something like, 'That poor kid being raised by two faggots.'"—Stuart sees there are many advantages for a child being raised by two dads or two moms: "They become more compassionate to differences in the world. The most important thing to teach a child is kindness. What a wonderful world that would be if every parent, whether mother and father, dad and dad, or mom and mom, taught their kids just that one thing."

Copie (Short for "Co-Parent")

Mary and her partner, Jane, raised their son Todd together. When he was young, he made up the name "Copie" for Jane as his co-parent. He called her that name until he was eight and realized he didn't want to address her that way in public; he was at the age where it becomes more important for a kid *not* to be different in the public eye, and so from that point on, he addressed her by her first name. For Todd, it was more an issue of not having a dad than of having two moms. Mary explained that she soon discovered her son was constantly being called "faggot" by one particular kid at school (we'll call him Dick). When Mary met Dick's mom, and Dick's mom found out Todd had two moms, Dick's mom said to Mary, "Oh, now I know why my son calls your son a faggot—it's because he has two moms." Mary told me she was left speechless. She felt there was nothing meaningful to say to someone who believed it was okay for their son to call her son a faggot because he had two moms.

Mary made a great point in saying that gay people are a minority raised by a non-minority and aren't visible. But then, if we have kids, they are automatically deemed part of a minority family.

I asked Mary what some advantages are for a kid who has same-sex parents. She said, "We have never become parents by accident. It is always a planned commitment. It's a more child-focused scenario." She added, "LGBTQ parents in general tend to be more involved in the day-to-day activities of their children and more emotionally in tune with them because of this, as well. It also gives kids awareness that you can be who you are."

Can You Miss Something You Never Had?

Many people worry that a child with two moms or two dads might be missing out by not having a mother or a father. I believe this is a legitimate concern. In a perfect world, every child should have positive male and female role models, but the best we can ask in this real world is for a child to be brought up with love and taught to be kind and to respect others. Whether a child is raised by a single mom or dad, a mom and a stepdad, grandparents, or two dads or two moms, love and strong values are what matter most. As a child of a traditional family, it took me a while to come to that conclusion. My only suggestion—which really comes from those I interviewed—is that if a child has same-sex parents, it might be good to have a friend or godparent of the other sex to be there as a role model as well.

In the book *Now That You Know: What Every Parent Should Know about Homosexuality*, by Betty Fairchild and Nancy Hayward, the authors highlighted many advantages for children of same-sex parents. One woman they interviewed about female same-sex parents stated, "There are things that a father would miss that the second mother picks up every time." Their research did not turn up any evidence that heterosexual parents are "better" parents in terms of offering love, support, or stability in the home.

Tips from COLAGE Literature on Children Talking about Their Nontraditional Families:

Children Ages Four to Seven
"Why doesn't Maria have a mother and father?"
As children go off to school, they become aware of other families. Other adults might approach these questions from a "deficit model," assuming that the

child is missing a parent. Instead, the children may just be noticing and wanting to talk about similarities and differences. For them, family configurations are a matter of fact. They do not naturally attach value to a particular kind of family.

Children want to talk about their families. They define and redefine their own families to include people, pets, and toys. They may even pretend to have brothers, sisters, and extra parents or ask you to pretend that you are someone else in relationship to them. They are just playing. They are not trying to change who is in their family or be anyone else. It is important for adults to recognize this as play and to respond in a way that is playful and matter-of-fact.

"I was born far away and my daddies brought me here to live with them."
Children are fascinated by stories of themselves as babies. They may be driven to share their life stories, including stories about adoption and conception. They may ask to hear these stories over and over again and will share them with friends, schoolmates, or anyone who will listen. Be aware that everything you tell them will potentially be shared with others. Having photo albums or baby books that document their life in your family helps them reinforce their sense of belonging and understand their relationships. We play an important role by giving them words to talk about their experiences and relationships.

(continued)

Donor (Alternative) Insemination
Sometimes adults have a hard time discussing things like donor insemination. Preparing simple answers ahead of time to the questions you know are coming can help you feel more comfortable, such as: "Your mommy and I wanted to have a baby. You grew from a special people egg in Mommy's body in a place called a womb." If pressed further, you can discuss the introduction of sperm by saying, "We also needed a seed from a man, which is called sperm, to help the egg grow into a baby. Our doctor helped us find someone who wanted to help us make a baby. The seed and egg grew to be you."

Family Equality Council Excerpts on Children Talking about Their Nontraditional Families:
Children Eight and Older
"Nobody talks about their parents."
For many children in the preadolescent and adolescent years, fitting in and being part of a group may be the most important thing. Around seven years old, some children no longer want or know how to talk about their families. This is especially true if their family is perceived to be "different." At this time, children also may need to be in charge of who they come out to about their family. Children often only share the

intimate details of their lives with a few close friends. They will learn where, when, and with whom it is safe to talk about their lives. When this occurs, many parents feel like their child is rejecting them or is ashamed of their sexuality or gender identity. Most of this behavior, however, is typical. In fact, heterosexual parents may also experience a sense of rejection for other reasons.

"Everyone uses 'gay' as an insult and the teachers don't say anything."
It is common for children in this age group to begin to call each other names like "gay," "faggot," "lezzy," and "dyke." Children recognize and are sensitive to attacks on people who are like the people in their families and communities. Our children often feel personally insulted when this name-calling occurs, even if it was not directed at them or their family. Parents can work with school systems to sensitize them to the impact of insulting language on their children. If this is not possible, parents can still talk to their children about their experiences and feelings and acknowledge how difficult this may be for them. Talking about the words, their meanings, and the ways in which they feel hurtful to us in our community helps children identify their own feelings about this kind of name-calling. It is important to help children separate their personal response to the name-calling from the intent on the part of the aggressor. In all cases, hurtful

(continued)

name-calling is wrong and our children can be helped to understand this.

"Some kids asked me if my mom is a lesbian. I don't know what to do."
This can be a scary time for our children. They need us to give them strategies for responding to the questions or insults of other children. Some strategies that have worked for children in this age group include:

• *Giving Direct Responses Such As "Yes, She Is"*
Children have reported that this takes the power away from the child asking the question. If the child tries to keep it a secret, other children can use it to tease or bully him or her. If they are honest and matter-of-fact, the words may lose their power.
• *Making a Joke in Response*
Some children feel more comfortable redirecting the questions or insults using humor. This may help children by getting them the approval of their peer group.
They also do not have to directly confirm or deny the comment.

• *Ignoring Comments*
Walking away from potentially inflammatory situations suits the personality of some children. They choose not to engage in discussions or confrontations. However, this may increase the teasing later on or cause them to worry about the next time it happens. These children may need

additional help with strategies or may need their parents to communicate with the school.

• *Finding a Supportive Group of Friends*
For all children, this is a time where having one or more close friends who can be trusted makes them feel safer. Allies are important. Parents can try to encourage children to find friends who will be accepting of their families. Children begin to seek out friends who they perceive to be the same as themselves. Groups such as COLAGE can offer local peer groups or a pen pal so children have contact with others who have similar families and experiences.

Concluding thoughts from Family Equality Council on children talking about their families: As children grow in their knowledge and understanding of the world and issues of race, sexual orientation, relationships, gender identity, and expression, their questions can become far more explicit. For example, they might ask:

"Did you know you were gay before you met Ray?"
"How did you choose the donor?"
"Why did you go to China to adopt me?"
"Why did you decide to become a woman? Do you not like men?"

Parents need to be careful not to read too much into their questions and use these as opportunities to educate their children about the full range of options available for

(continued)

creating families and expressing identity. The best way to teach this is to tell your own personal story or stories of others you know. Read your child's cues for how much he or she can handle at each given moment. It is fine to offer some information and wait for them to come back for greater clarity or detail when they are ready.

CHAPTER 4

Transgender: "Kids, Your Dad, Well, She Has Something to Tell You"

I was encouraged by Robin Marquis, the former national program director at COLAGE, to include a chapter on transgender people, and I realize the importance of doing so. In recent years, I've heard other gay people make oppositional comments such as, "Who decided to add transgender to the gay community?" I've found their attitude a bit odd, because although transgender people are different from gay people in many ways, they do go through so many similar struggles such as identity issues, being different, discrimination, and trying to be accepted by others.

When I started this book, I knew very little about trans people and had only met a few. Several years ago, I saw the film *Transamerica*, about a preoperative male-to-female transsexual who finds out that she fathered a son who is now a teenage runaway, hustling on the streets of New York. Although the film helped to bring transgender issues into the spotlight, and Felicity Huffman won a Golden Globe and an Independent Spirit award for her awesome portrayal, some transgender people were ticked off that a real transgender person didn't play the role. I can see how that could be upsetting. What I also found upsetting was that Dolly Parton (whom I'm a huge fan of) didn't win the Oscar for "Travelin' Thru," the song she wrote for the film's soundtrack, which was nominated for an Academy Award for Best Song. (The Oscar instead went to "It's Hard out Here for a Pimp.") In all seriousness, to the issue of who the role went to, perhaps filmmakers should consider transgender people playing the roles of transgender people? I really enjoyed *Transamerica* because it helped me develop a better understanding of transgender people.

The documentary *In My Shoes* features a candid interview with a girl who was being raised by her uncle (who was born female). She tells a story about how one of her friends reacted when she saw an old picture of her uncle when he had been a woman. The friend freaked out and simply couldn't handle the concept of a person changing genders. Perhaps it's not so much about people being unaccepting but more that we aren't taught enough about what transgenderism really means. Many people simply don't understand it and aren't accustomed to seeing people different from themselves (except maybe on TV), so they're extremely uncomfortable when they do. The only way to surpass these barriers is with more informed discussions and more movies, TV shows, and books bringing these issues into popular culture so they're not so foreign. Some have already tried to do just that, such as *Boys Don't Cry* in 1999, for which

Hilary Swank won the Oscar for Best Actress, and *Dallas Buyers Club* in 2013, featuring Jared Leto's 2014 Oscar-winning role as a transgender woman. There was another highly acclaimed film that introduced a transgender character way back when I was in high school. In 1982, *The World According to Garp* starred Robin Williams in one of his first major film roles after leaving the TV series *Mork and Mindy*. The film featured John Lithgow, who gave an amazing performance as a transgender ex-football player, Roberta Muldoon.

As I mentioned, I had very limited knowledge of the transgender community before writing this book; conducting research for this chapter was a great learning experience for me. Hopefully these examples of transgender people and their struggles will give people more of an insight and understanding of them, so it will be easier for them to come out and to continue to have good relationships with their children.

Coming Out Gradually

Kendall Evans is a transgender woman and a California licensed marriage and family therapist specializing in violence and abuse. I met her at a PFLAG meeting. She was there with her father and son. She said to the group, "I am not changing from being a man to being a woman, I am changing from living as a man to living as myself." Her coming out and transitioning was a gradual process that began very late in life (her late fifties, in fact). She explained how she always felt different through her entire life and couldn't quite place it. Although her son had been a little apprehensive about her transition at first, he is now very supportive and certainly enjoys the fact he got a whole new wardrobe out of it (all Kendall's male clothes). Kendall believes that a gradual process of "coming out" as transgender is probably better for most people, although her father and son both had some solid indicators with her shopping habits. "After watching you shop, you're a woman," her father joked, referring to how long she took in the stores. But they had also noticed the gradual change in her preferences as well: Kendall's wardrobe also became more and more feminine as time went by.

By the time she came out, Kendall's son was in his late teens and already out of school, so they didn't have to deal with any issues there. However, she still strongly encouraged him to read the PFLAG brochures about transgender people and the literature for the children of transgender parents. She said it helped him a lot. "It's important for kids and adults to go out of their way to try to understand [each other], and going to family therapy was very helpful too," Kendall explained.

Speaking with Kendall was as much of a learning experience as watching the documentaries and movies that taught me about transgendered people. For example, she told me that some people are bi-gender, depending on the day or time of day. In other words, some days they feel more like a man and some days more like a woman. These feelings can even shift through different parts of the same day as well.

She also told me about Lana Wachowski, the transgender codirector of *The Matrix* and *Cloud Atlas*. Lana had received an HRC (Human Rights Campaign) award in the past, and her acceptance speech had a profound effect on Kendall. After our interview, I immediately went home and watched the speech online and found it extremely moving. Lana's powerful message was that she was being awarded for "being herself," saying, "This moment is fulfilling the cathartic arc of rejection to acceptance without ever integrating the pathology of a society who refuses to acknowledge the spectrum of gender in the exact same blind way they refuse to see a spectrum of race or sexuality." Lana's sister Lilly (formally Andrew), who works with Lana cowriting and codirecting many films, is also a trans woman, which makes their professional partnership—as well as their familial relationship—pretty rare.

Kendall also told me about a recent health scare that required her son to call an ambulance for her. He went along to the hospital and made sure they got all the pronouns right on the paperwork. Anywhere it said "he," her son made sure it was changed to "she." Apparently, he did such a thorough job that a short time later, Kendall received a letter in the mail from their insurance company, informing her that she was overdue for her Pap smear.

You Are Not Like Other Kids

A friend of mine referred me to Daralyn (Dal) Maxwell, a transgender woman. I interviewed her by phone from my home in sunny California, where it was about seventy degrees, while she was in Freeport, Maine, trying to stay warm in freezing temperatures. We had a very interesting conversation and had a lot more to talk about than the weather. Dal is a volunteer DJ for the community radio station WMPG, where she has a weekly program of LGBT-centric news and contemporary Celtic music. She is also a former board member of SAGE (Services and Advocacy for GLBT Elders), which is an organization that improves the quality of life for older LGBTQ adults in Maine, and a former board member of the Maine Transgender Network.

She recalled a memory of a cold, gray November afternoon in the late 1950s when she was a five-year-old boy watching *Howdy Doody*. She said it suddenly felt like the universe welled up inside of her head and shouted, "YOU ARE NOT LIKE OTHER KIDS." It would be years before she understood the context and significance of that.

Dal is active at a synagogue where about 10 percent of the congregation is LGBT. When she first went there, she asked how they felt about transgender people and they said, "Who are we to judge?" Before that, it had been a long time since she had attended a synagogue. In fact, she said that shortly before her bar mitzvah back in the mid-1960s, she had told her parents she couldn't go through with it, and they canceled. The real reason was she couldn't be part of any ceremony where she'd have to say, "I am now a man." This story made me wonder if there were other children who knew they were transgender at a very young age and if they actually changed a bar mitzvah to a bat mitzvah or vice versa.

And, of course, I decided to do more research and did find an article in *Jewish News Syndicate* from January 2016 by Maayan Jaffe-Hoffman, which tells of Rabbi Eric Gurvis, senior rabbi of Temple Shalom in Newton, Massachusetts, performing a handful of bar and bat mitzvah ceremonies for transgender boys and girls. Instead of naming the ceremony a bar or bat mitzvah, Gurvis called it a "mitzvah journey to becoming a responsible adult Jew." The synagogue removed the bar/bat mitzvah label from the certificate that it gave the teenager. I'm sure there are other examples of this elsewhere, but this was a great find.

Fairly direct and outspoken on matters of being trans, Dal said her opinion is that "Transition ain't for pussies." She also said, "Transitioning people are often self-absorbed, rarely talk about real feelings, and don't like to be looked at as weak. Transitioning is modification to bring congruence between core identity and physical presence." Her advice on transitioning: "Act with common sense, integrity, common good, and betterment of yourself."

Daralyn is the father of two children who are now adults (her daughter was eight years old and her son was five when they were told), but Daralyn is now estranged from them because her ex's anger was so profound she worked hard to emotionally alienate and disenfranchise the kids from Dal—and it worked. She says she did have one or two discussions with them while they were still talking. Her daughter was tough to talk to because they had a terrific bond before that and her "dad" was leaving. Daralyn assured her that everything was pretty much the same. Her son was even more difficult because he was two when they split up (the gender issue is not why they split up) and he fell under the "spell" of her ex. Daralyn's is another story of a spouse poisoning the child's relationship with the other parent. This happens in many divorces because of anger, but I think it happens more with gay people, and even more for transgender people. When adults act like kids, it's hard to have the conversations that need to be had with the kids.

Answering Kids' Questions About Transitioning

I spoke to a transgender woman in Arizona—we'll call her Phoenix—about how she deals with the questions kids ask about transitioning. Her advice was, "The shorter the answers, the better. Don't bombard them with too much information. Let them know they can ask more questions later if they want to.

Not a whole lot you need to tell." Phoenix also said that her own nieces and nephews had asked things like, "Are you going to have an operation?" Her answer was, "Maybe." They also asked other questions like, "Are we still gonna be together? What do I call you now? What does this mean for your marriage? Are you gonna dress like a woman; are you going to change your name?" These answers will vary on the individual but these are some questions you can expect.

Phoenix commented on how much easier it is for children to accept such information as opposed to some adults. She theorized that grown-ups often can't fathom different gender identities, or they are offended, or think they have certain moral standings. But with the younger generation, it is a nonissue. She also said that the many online support systems, through social media and groups like PFLAG, make things a lot easier now as well. People can realize they are not alone and that there are plenty of others going through the same things. Phoenix also does some work at PFLAG and told me how just a week prior to our interview, a mother had come in very distraught after learning that her child was transgender. Later, the woman left in high spirits, still trying to understand, but knowing that her child would be fine.

"We Already Know."

At another PFLAG meeting I attended, there were two guest speakers who were also a couple. Mike/Michelle identifies as transgender and Robin was bisexual. Although they hadn't met until they were in their sixties, they seemed to be soul mates. A few weeks after the meeting, I interviewed Mike/Michelle and I learned that she hadn't accepted her transgender identity until she was in her fifties. At her age, and in her physical condition, full physical transition was not deemed appropriate. There are a lot of transgender folks who, due to age/physical condition or financial matters, do not fully transition. She uses the name Mike/Michelle now in selected circles to generate questions, which allows others to see who a transgender person may be. In turn, that creates more "safe space" in the world for other transgender folks. She says, "We all have to do what we can to eliminate the killing of transgender people."

Mike/Michelle had previously been married, and although she and her wife did divorce, it was amicable and so was their approach to dealing with their children, who were both in their late teens at the time. They sat down with their son and daughter for a family meeting and Mike/Michelle started explaining about transgender people. But before she could say that she was transgender, the two kids said, "Dad, we already know."

Mike/Michelle was surprised and asked, "How did you know?" The son explained that once when he had been at home visiting from college, he needed to borrow a pair of shoes and went into his father's closet. He found a large woman's shoe as well as women's clothes that he knew wouldn't fit his mother.

Her daughter said that she had used her dad's computer once and saw all the bookmarks about transgender topics. At that point, Mike/Michelle didn't have much more to say to them besides: "If you want to learn more, you can come out with me when I am out as Michelle."

The son hesitated and said, "Let me think about it," but the daughter accepted the invite and asked, "When?" She ended up having a blast going with Mike/Michelle to drag shows where the DJ was also transgender. Although the son was a little uncomfortable at first, he came around fairly quickly and then also accompanied Mike/Michelle to various places in the transgender community. Mike/Michelle told an interesting story about one night when they were at the Queen Mary nightclub, where there were some male military personnel there dressed up as women. They were about to be sent to Iraq and explained their reason for going out that night by saying, "We don't want to die without ever experiencing this."

Now her children are grown, and Mike/Michelle has a twelve-year-old grandchild who is gender fluid (which means they do not identify as a fixed gender and prefer the pronoun "they"). The grandchild's parents and Mike/Michelle waited until the grandchild was eleven to have Grandpa Mike come out as Grandma Michelle and explain it to them. Mike/Michelle is out to all of her partner Robin's family, including Robin's ten-year-old niece, who asked questions like, "Are you a boy or a girl?" To which Mike/Michelle responded, "Kind of both." The niece simply said, "That's interesting." The niece has also seen her both as Mike and as Michelle and asked, "What is it like being Michelle?" Mike/Michelle answered, "It's a lot of work."

Mike/Michelle also addressed people who struggle with accepting transgender people or question whether the lifestyle is right or wrong. Mike/Michelle said, "It's just a characteristic, like a size 10 shoe. It just is, so live and let live."

Progressive Parenting

My good friend Marti sent me this heartwarming story about her son, Billy.

While Billy was in kindergarten, his best friend was a boy named James, who at the time I suspected may be transgender, which later proved to be true. One day, about midway through the school year, Billy asked me if James was a boy or a girl—because as he told me, "He likes My Little Pony." Billy seemed worried. So I told him that all that really matters about who you are is how you feel on the inside and that boys and girls sometimes like all kinds of stuff. Billy told me the other kids might make fun of his new backpack and then he might cry. So I said, "Well, if anybody does that, it's not nice." I told him that if anybody makes fun of James's new backpack, to tell them to be nice to James because he's allowed to like whatever he wants to and not to make fun of his friend because hurting people's feelings is mean.

Then we talked about colors and how there is no such thing as "boy colors" and "girl colors," that it's just something that people made up. Our conversation ended with him telling me not to worry because James was his best friend and best friends look out for each other. About a month or two later, while walking home from school hand in hand with James on our way to one of our many playdates, Billy said to both James and me, "People always say 'boys will be boys' but they should say 'girls can be boys too' because they can—it only matters how you feel on the inside." During this rather proud Momma moment, I looked at James for his reaction and saw his smile beaming from ear to ear. I smiled, too, and said, 'That's true, Billy, girls can be boys and boys can be girls too." Billy looked at me and said, "It sure is a crazy, mixed up world—but also it's awesome because you can just be whoever you want to be."

I think it's great that Marti was open to these kinds of conversations with her son at such an early age. She also showed how accepting she was of everyone and was teaching her child to be that way, too, which also encourages him to be true to himself.

Excerpts from COLAGE Transition Tips for Parents

"See the transition as not being about the [parent] going through change, but the whole family going through change. Everyone needs support."
—Steve Vinay G., age 48

Coming out to family is a major issue for transgender people and can be a difficult process. Please keep in mind that the entire family transitions, not just the transgender parent. Every member of the family needs time and support to adjust to the changes of a gender transition. The process of acceptance can take a while and is often ongoing. You should make sure that your children know—through language and action—that no matter what, you will still be their parent.

As a parent, remember that your children come first and your transition comes second. Transition is an inherently self-focused process as you align your body and appearance with your gender identity. The best way to be a responsible parent during transition is to make your children a major priority throughout the process. Sometimes this means that you have to compromise your ideal time frame for your transition in order to keep relationships with your family healthy. We suggest working with a transgender-competent therapist to deal with your own issues before coming out to your kids. The more comfortable you are with your decision, the easier it will be to answer their questions and support them through your transition. How you tell your children is critical. Try to avoid coming out around the holidays or major family events, when there is often extra pressure and expectations. You can have the conversation in a safe space with plenty of time, where the conversation can't be overheard, and where they will feel comfortable continuing the conversation.

Knowing your kids and the way they process will help you decide just what to say. If you are nervous, you can write it down first or practice with a friend. Come out to them in an age-appropriate way that fits with their personality. It's best to keep your sentences short and concise to avoid overwhelming them with too much information (such as details about surgeries or hormones). People's responses will vary—some children will ask a million questions and others will have no reaction at all. Keep in mind that they may not want to talk about it right away or may just want some space to think things over. Regardless of their initial reaction, you can make yourself available for future conversations.

Many times, this is a traumatic event in that it changes the way your child sees the world. Throughout the transition, it's important to acknowledge that this is a process for everyone and that feelings are okay. If possible, you and your spouse/partner (or ex-spouse/ex-partner) should create a united front to support your children through your transition, especially if you are

(continued)

separating or divorcing. Continue to be a responsible,
caring parent and remind them that you will love them
no matter what.

You can also provide your children with transitional
objects, such as a letter or card, something they can
hold on to to remind them that you will always be their
parent. Children benefit when you involve them as
much as possible. Try to give them advance notice about
decisions you are making and how they may impact your
appearance, your day-to-day lives, or your family. When
possible, make some decisions together. Respect your
children's wishes about how, when, and to whom they
come out to about you. We encourage you to give them a
say about what to call you and how involved you will be
in their public lives. If the decisions your child is making
about these issues are hard for you, discuss your feelings
with other adults, trans parents, or therapists, rather than
expecting your child to take care of you.

Your child may benefit from additional support
throughout your transition. You can provide them
with options of other supportive adults to talk with,
such as a therapist or family friend. Encourage them to
connect with other people with LGBTQ parents through
COLAGE—either locally or through the internet. As
a parent, you can help them understand that there is so
much difference in the world and everyone is explaining
their own difference. Ultimately, that is the gift of having
a transgender parent. Visit www.colage.org to connect
your children with other people with trans parents

through a local COLAGE chapter or our virtual online chapter. Request a copy of the official KOT (Kids of Trans) Resource Guide and access their other resources for LGBTQ parents and their children. Contact the KOT program: kidsoftrans@colage.org.

COLAGE *Literature about Challenges for Kids of Transgender Parents*

The following discusses the different challenges kids of transgender parents face as opposed to kids of gay or lesbian parents. Here are some excerpts:

Sexual Orientation vs. Gender Identity: A parent's sexual orientation and a parent's gender identity impact their children in different ways. (For example, if I am in public with my gay parent, people may not know that they are gay. Whereas if I am in public with my transgender parent, people may suspect that their gender expression differs from their assigned sex.)

Societal Awareness and Acceptance: Gay, lesbian, bisexual, and queer people have made incredible progress over the last few decades in increasing visibility and acceptance in society. Transgender people have also made progress, but have been less visible and less accepted than

(continued)

gay and lesbian people. While transgender people are becoming more visible, the fact that they have children is less widely known.

Legal Protections: Gay, lesbian, bisexual, and queer people have more legal protections than transgender people. Depending on the state, transgender parents can also face immense challenges in court custody cases, leaving children vulnerable to being taken away from or legally estranged from a parent.

Transition: Many people with transgender parents witness their parent's transition from one gender to another . . . As we witness our parent change their gender, we may grieve the loss of our parent's former self. We struggle with understanding and/or reestablishing our relationship to our parent as they become who they need to be. As KOTs (Kids of Trans), we are often forced to hear or answer invasive questions about the medical processes, genitalia, or other details about our parents.

Transphobia in the LGBTQ Community: As people with transgender parents, KOTs often encounter transphobia in the world. Sometimes lesbian, gay, bisexual, or queer people are transphobic toward our families or other transgender people. Just because someone is LGBQ (or has an LGB/Q parent) does not necessarily mean that they understand transgender issues.

After interviewing a few transgender people and reading the books and seeing the films they recommended, I have a much better understanding than I did before. It made me realize just how painful it must be to feel so strongly that you must fully become the gender you feel you are despite the possible ridicule, risk of losing all your friends and family, and, in some cases life-threatening danger. I strongly encourage everyone to learn more about what they don't know and to try to understand people who are different from themselves. People are afraid of the unknown. Wouldn't the world be a better place if we all got to know each other and live and let live?

CHAPTER 5

Kids Say the Darndest Things

Since this book is essentially about kids and their acceptance of the LGBTQ community, it was imperative for me to get their perspective as well. The following are some questions I asked children (some now grown) with LGBTQ relatives and their various responses about their experiences.

Were there any issues or interesting stories (serious, humorous, or heartwarming) at school or other social settings regarding having one or more gay, lesbian, bisexual, or transgender parent(s) (relative[s])?

- **Amanda:** I wasn't necessarily embarrassed of my mom up through middle school but that was the age when kids (especially boys) were becoming very mean, so I was very on guard about my home life. Once high school started, however, many of my friends knew, and I was very open and proud about my family, though, to my hometown's credit, I never encountered a peer who expressed distaste toward my family.

- **Trevor:** The only issue I had at school was that when some people heard that I had a gay parent, they automatically assumed that I was also gay, but I'm not. This wasn't offensive to me or anything, it was more bothersome that they would stereotype and assume something without question just to be mean.

If you could give advice to other kids who have a gay/lesbian/ bisexual/transgender parent or relative, what would it be?

- **Sam:** I would tell them to accept the blessing they have been given. Yes, I believe I am blessed to have a gay father. It truly has made me the person I am today in the most positive way. Always embrace your family and never be bullied into silence.
- **Carla:** Don't think of your family or your parents as being different. For me, my moms were always just my parents and nothing else. If your family is happy, you're luckier than many others out there, whether anyone is heterosexual, homosexual, or whatever else.

- **Jamie:** I'd say to them to always remember you are lucky. You are growing up in a home or around others who are full of love and acceptance. Whoever you are will never be questioned or an issue. And you will easily be more accepting and openhearted to anyone you meet, something many people lack the ability to do. Love is love no matter what shape or form. Love and support your relative the most you can and they will do the same for you.

- **Huck:** You don't need to prove anything. Be yourself. When I was growing up with a gay dad, I felt a need to prove my masculinity and strength. I realize now, I didn't.

What are some benefits of having an LGBTQ parent or relative, or same-sex parents?

- **Natalia:** The biggest benefit I think is how accepting and open-minded I've become because of how I was brought up. I'm also very thankful for every family member I've gained from it.

- **Joe:** It gives you an amazing perspective of the world around you and you realize everyone is different. I learned I don't need to fit into a box, I can be who I am, it's all okay. Because of my gay mom, I think I feel compassion for all and try to be kind to everyone, including those who are different or who I don't understand.

What else can you tell us about your family and personal experience?

- **Cameron:** After my parents divorced, my mom met a woman she was with for only about a year. Then she met another woman with two twin boys the same age as my brother. They were together for almost ten years but unfortunately called it quits. But I've stayed in contact, and will continue to always, with her ex and her ex's sons. She will always be a mother to me and her sons will always be my brothers. She's also married to a new woman now who I also consider a mother (and she considers me a daughter). I have four moms and I couldn't be more thankful for each of them. My biological mother is still dating around. I hope she finds a new serious partner soon so she can be happy and won't be so alone at home.

- **Vanessa:** My biological parents divorced when I was seven years old, and my mother began dating women while my father soon met my stepmother, who he married within a few years. My biological mom was with a woman who lived with us for ten years, and she quickly became another mother figure to me. They split around the time I was eighteen or nineteen, but I continue to think of my biological mom's ex as one of my mothers, and she is now happily married to her wife, who she met a few years ago. So, to break it down: biological dad happily married to stepmom; two moms happily married; biological mom currently dating.

Did you see any movies or read any books on this subject that were helpful? What were they and how did they help?

- **Ellie:** I don't remember any movies or books in particular, but I do have fond memories of watching the *Ellen* show and *Rosie O'Donnell Show* with my mom growing up. It was just something nice that we'd actually spend time doing together.
- **Peter:** We watched a lot of *Will & Grace*. It was one of our weekly family rituals, and it was definitely nice to feel represented on TV.

How old were you when you found out your parent or relative was LGBT? How did you find out, or how were you told? How did you react?

- **Matthias:** I was six or seven years old. After my parents divorced, my mother began a relationship with a woman. I don't remember how I was initially told, but I was okay with it from the start. It was probably explained to me that sometimes men love men, and sometimes women love women (as was the case with my mother).
- **Indiana:** I was very little when I realized it. It wasn't so much that I remember being told but became aware and accepting of it. My parents divorced when I was around four years old and soon after my mom started seeing a woman who had two kids as well. Nothing seemed weird or unusual.

- **Caroline Shores, daughter of Del Shores:** I was two years old when my father came out. I can't recall how I was told or how I reacted because I don't think a two-year-old can really understand a concept that big. But because I was so young, it's all I ever knew and that is exactly the reason I am the way I am: accepting and understanding of all types of people.

Growing up with an LGBT parent

Caroline Shores: Proud Daughter of Gay Dad

In addition to participating in the survey, Caroline Shores, daughter of Del Shores, was also kind enough to sit down with me and share her experience growing up with a gay father. For Caroline, "gay" was always around. Her father came out when she was barely a toddler, and she went to a very progressive elementary school in California, where she never had any problems since several other students had gay/lesbian parents.

In her words: "When I was twelve or thirteen, I went to middle school in Van Nuys, California, and that was the first time I started to see homophobia. My first experience with that was when I was having a slumber party for my thirteenth birthday. One of the girls told me yes, she was coming. A couple days later she said, 'I'm sorry, but my dad won't let me go because your dad is gay.' I didn't even know why that was an issue. It didn't make sense to me. I went kind of ballistic on her, really huge fight, and [for the] first time ever, I felt hatred toward my family.

"It continued in that middle school. Students used expressions like 'That's so gay.' Students called each other faggots. I would tell the principal and she would then have a lot of tolerance talks with the students. These kids were very rough. My next experience was in Spanish class. We had a family tree exercise and in my family tree I had my stepdad and my dad on the same side and had that written in Spanish. The teacher said during her presentation, 'Oh, I think you got confused. That goes on the other side next to your mom.' I go, 'No, that's my dad's husband,' and this kid, a boy (sorry, boys, but the consensus is boys are worse than girls when it comes to this) started making these really graphic comments in the back, like 'faggot this' and sexual comments. I stopped the presentation and said, 'Can you come up and tell me that to my face?'

"He said, 'You heard what I said,' and I said, 'No, come up and tell me to my face.' The teacher was like, 'Just continue,' I'm like 'No, let him come up and tell me to my face.'

"She made me go to the principal's office.

"She didn't really hear the boy. She just saw and heard me arguing with him. The principal suspended him. His mom called my mom and said, 'We didn't raise him that way, we're sorry.' There were consequences. It was shocking to me. I was blind to that kind of attitude.

"The progression in the last few years has been huge. Now, probably other people would have stood up for me, too, in that situation. It's not acceptable anywhere. Best thing to do with bullies is stand up for yourself; they don't like that. They want to pick on the weak. This is my family and I want to stand up for them. It's an obligation, it's not a choice. And it's nothing to be ashamed of."

I also asked Caroline about her experiences with being a child of LGBTQ parents and practicing a religion. She said, "I think that's where the hatred really starts, with religion and what's taught. I went to a Catholic school. I had a problem with one of the teachers who was so homophobic. In a private Catholic school, they can really do whatever they want. We have to sign a contract so the rules are different. I fought back and pulled out my evidence. Lately when I hear anything religious based and homophobic, I try to keep in mind these people are on the wrong side of history. They are the ones who are going to be looking stupid in the future. I chalk it up to ignorance, not knowing what they are talking about. It's easier not to be offended this way because they don't know any better and you really can't change everyone."

Another subject Caroline has had to school people on, besides religion, is the "It's a choice" argument. Here's how she handled it: "I have a male friend who inquired whether another male friend had a girlfriend, and I said, 'No, he has a boyfriend.' He said, 'Whatever, it's a phase.' I go, 'It's not a phase,' but he was like, 'I mean, he's choosing it,' and he was so adamant about it. So finally, I asked him, 'Okay. When did you choose to be straight?' He was like, 'Yeah, you have a point.' A lot of the time that question does the trick of making people understand it is not a choice. Why would you want your rights taken away from you?"

When we discussed the benefits of having a gay dad, she said she considered it a blessing. "I wouldn't be the person I am today without it. My dad has always been my rock, the person I look up to. Because I was two when my dad came out, my view of the world was always acceptance, always love. I was always prone to be friends with anyone different, like the nerdy kid or the kid who had no friends. It made me more accepting to everyone. I don't know if I would have been that way otherwise."

Caroline also made a good point about how much easier it's becoming for gay people to come out, find support groups, and not feel as alone with so many online resources and social media providing immediate access to information. "There's even a white rapper, Macklemore, with a gay anthem song [with Ryan Lewis] called 'Same Love,'" she said. Since the hip-hop industry has been known for not being very gay-friendly, Caroline saw it as a huge step for a straight rapper to come out with a song like this. "That wouldn't have happened even a few years ago. So much progress is being made." Sure enough, a few months after our interview, Macklemore performed "Same Love" on the Grammys telecast as Queen Latifah married same-sex couples and Madonna joined in with "Open Your Heart." Caroline Shores is a wise and loving young woman, living proof that gay or not gay, Del Shores is an excellent parent.

Mandy: Gay Parents Won't Make You Gay

I interviewed a nineteen-year-old girl from New York—we'll call her Mandy. Mandy had two gay mothers and a gay dad, although she was mostly raised by her two moms. For anyone concerned that a child is more prone to being gay if raised by gay parents, well, Mandy had three gay parents and still turned out straight.

Mandy emphasized how important it is that same-sex parents take more time to discuss with their kids what they may encounter at school and how some kids may react to them having a family that is a little bit different. Mandy said that during her own years at elementary school, she found people were more confused about her family than anything, and she remembers having to explain things over and over. She also remembers some of the kids and parents weren't very cool with it and simply felt it wasn't normal. In fourth grade, some students even told her that her family was messed up. Of course, such comments really hurt her, but Mandy said that she was lucky that her teacher and the school were very supportive of her family and made efforts to deal with the kids who were bullying her throughout the years from third to sixth grade. However, she also admitted that she learned to be ambiguous about her parents and to even lie about her last name, dropping the hyphen. Sometimes she even told people she just had a mom and a dad like everyone else. In high school, Mandy felt more comfortable being open about her family and she said that she was lucky to grow up somewhere less conservative than other places. At nineteen, she is now able to be open about her family, but she told me about a friend who also has a gay parent who lives in a small town and has spent her entire life lying about her family because of the conservative community there.

Mandy also brought up another important concern for kids of LGBTQ parents: there's more pressure on the children of gay parents to be less problematic, or to do better in school—to basically be more "perfect"—because they are often poster children. If they are not perfect, some may be quick to pass judgment and point a finger, saying, "See! Children should not be raised by two moms or two dads. They should be raised by a mother and father." Mandy said as hard as it may be for some kids to ignore this kind of pressure, they must remember that they aren't poster children for anyone but themselves. "It's important that the kids know that the family doesn't have to be perfect because *no family is perfect*, and they don't have to be a perfect child because that is not possible for human beings. That is a lot of pressure to be put on the kids, so it is important to speak with them on these issues."

Mandy also mentioned that kids should be prepared for the fact that many people will ask inappropriate and invasive questions, often things that they wouldn't even think to ask of straight families. She explained that although she has mostly tried to answer such questions, it's also important to let people know when the questions are not appropriate. Being a child of same-sex parents does not mean you have less of a right to privacy than everyone else.

When I asked her if she experienced some benefits to being raised by two moms, Mandy said, "It taught me a lot about relationships." She explained that her parents are in an equal relationship, independent to stand on their own, yet they take care of each other. Mandy said it's exactly what she wants in a relationship with a man: equal rights. She learned from her moms that she can be independent and doesn't have to put up with typical boys or needing anyone to protect her. Mandy said she wants a boy to take care of and she wants to be taken care of as well. She also talked about her gay dad and how she loves that he is strong but not in a way that relies on his masculinity; he is a good example of why it's wrong that many parents feel the need to push gender roles on their kids. Even today, there is still a common false perception that boys and girls have to be and act in certain ways.

Mandy also told me about her dad's brother, who is very conservative and not completely okay with him being gay. Her uncle also has kids, and one of them is a boy who has always adored Mandy's father. In fact, when the boy was seven, he announced, "I want to be gay." Although he had really just been expressing his love for his uncle and how he wanted to be like him, Mandy said that her cousin's parents' jaws had dropped in horror when he said this. The story speaks to another very good point Mandy brought up: Some people are okay with their sibling or cousin or someone they know being gay, but if one of their kids were to be gay, it would be a whole different story. I believe that even superstar Cher had this issue. She had many gay friends and is loved by a huge gay fan base, but she had trouble when her daughter Chastity came out as a lesbian and then later as transgender, changing his name to Chaz. If a parent truly wants to be a good parent, then they should be okay with whatever their child turns out to be as long as it's not harming others. Perhaps a good question everyone should ask themselves even before they become a parent is, Would I be okay with my son or daughter being gay?

A "Kids Say the Darndest Things" Moment

The following is an excerpt from Rip Corley's book *The Final Closet: The Gay Parents' Guide for Coming Out to Their Children*. It is a conversation between a seven-year-old and his gay dad:

Kid: "Do you make love with the man you live with the way you and Mommy did?"
Dad: "Yes."
Kid: "Isn't that against the law?"
Dad: "Not anymore."
Kid: "Good, I wouldn't want you to get in trouble."

Son of a Transgender Woman and How
He Came to Accept it

In addition to interviewing Kendall Evans for chapter 4, I also had the opportunity to speak with her son, Ben, who was twenty-one at the time. Ben admitted that when his dad told him the news about being transgender, it was a little hard to accept. In fact, one of the first things he said to his dad was, "I'm not gonna be seen with you if you're wearing a dress!" Ben says that he wasn't angry and he didn't hate his dad or anything, he just didn't understand. It didn't make sense to him. Even his grandma had said about his dad, "He was just doing it to get attention or to try something new," although Kendall had been in his fifties at the time and it was unlikely that he would act out like a teenager and do something drastic simply to get attention. There are certainly people who will do pretty much anything to get attention, but having a sex change operation isn't one of them.

Ben said that, gradually, he was able to accept that his dad was transgender. He also realized that there had been some previous signs before his dad came out. For example, he noticed his dad seemed very interested in transgender books and films. Unfortunately, Ben's mom still does not accept the situation at all and told him never to call his dad "Mom." She doesn't want people to think she is a lesbian.

I asked Ben what advice he would give to other kids of a transgender person, and he said, "It could be worse." A simple statement, but I think it's the best way to look at almost any issue or problem you may think you have in the grand scheme of things. He also added a strong message for everyone to keep in mind: "Accept people for who they are as opposed to who you want them to be."

CHAPTER 6

School
(Jeers To Peers Who Bully Queers)

School is not an easy place to be different. It's not even an easy place to be the same, especially during the middle school and high school years. School is where all kinds of jokes are told, including gay jokes. Some kids can be cruel. and most kids are extremely sensitive when it comes to their peers. How do these gay jokes affect young LGBTQ people and those still struggling with their sexuality or identity issues? How do these jokes affect kids with LGBTQ family members?

When I asked these very questions in my survey, many respondents indicated the phrase "That's so gay" was commonly used at school with a derogatory implication. One respondent said that his teenage nephew became so bothered by it that he eventually told his friends to stop using the expression because of its negative connotation. He explained to them that he had a gay uncle and that his uncle also happened to be pretty cool.

Even I have overheard my own nephew and niece use the expression once—their mom (my sister) immediately told them to stop doing so. Although I knew they really didn't mean any harm by it, I also realized the negative and contagious impact of kids hearing it used over and over.

Although many children of gay parents integrate the love from their families into their conduct, they can still be subject to outside influences and are often bombarded with messages that basically say being gay is bad, and that gay parents are unfit. They hear news reports about hate crimes and murders of LGBTQ people, as well as political debates about the legitimacy of civil rights for LGBTQ families.

Bullying is another big problem in schools all over the world. Although it's been more than seventeen years since the tragic death of Matthew Shepard, his brutal murder still has a major impact on the LGBTQ community. Matthew Shepard was a twenty-one-year-old student from Casper, Wyoming, who was savagely beaten to death by a group of violent bullies simply because he was gay.

In 2008, eighth grader Larry King was killed over his sexual orientation. A fellow student, fourteen-year-old Brandon McInerney, had shot Larry twice in the head because he found out Larry had a crush on him.

In 2009, eleven-year-old Carl Joseph Walker Hoover killed himself because the bullying and constant harassment he suffered at school became too much for him to bear. It was later reported that much of his suffering stemmed from constant comments like "You act gay" and "Are you gay?"

In 2010, yet another tragic death occurred, again illustrating the deadly consequences of even nonviolent forms of harassment. Tyler Clementi was an eighteen-year-old Rutgers University freshman when he jumped off a bridge, ending his own life. Classmates secretly recorded him on a webcam kissing another guy and then posted it online for all to see. Such brutality and bullying affects not only the victims themselves, but also kids with LGBTQ relatives. As long as bullying continues to exist, many of these kids fear that their loved ones could become the next victim.

The good news is that things are getting better, especially with more recent positive events, such as the coming out of high-profile professional athletes. In 2013, NBA pro basketball player Jason Collins became the first player still active in a major US professional sports league to announce that he is gay. While Collins hid his sexual orientation until 2013, he said he quietly made a statement for gay rights by wearing No. 98 with the Boston Celtics and the Washington Wizards. The number refers to 1998, the year Matthew Shepard was killed. It became one of the NBA's hottest-selling jerseys after he signed with the Nets in 2014.

We're getting there, but we've still got a ways to go. In the meantime, it's up to adults to have this discussion with kids, especially the kids with LGBTQ relatives who most likely have fears and concerns that need to be addressed. By being open, we can eventually turn the negative bias into real understanding and prevent these senseless tragedies from occurring.

Bully

The documentary *Bully* (2011) is an excellent film that examines peer-to-peer bullying in schools across the United States. It was directed by Lee Hirsch and written by Hirsch and Cynthia

Lowen. The DVD cover reads "A Movie Your Kids Must See," but I think it's something that everyone must see, not just kids. The film is very moving and deals with all kinds of bullying, whether the kids are introverted, overweight, or gay. One of the subjects of the film is a lesbian in a small, conservative town. When she came out, her parents had been very supportive, but every single one of her classmates at school had reacted by moving their chairs away from her. The neighbors, who had been friends of the parents for years, stopped talking to the family as well. It eventually became too much and the family decided to remove their daughter from the high school.

The book you're reading is for those very people who live in those very places and may need help dealing with extreme prejudice, or at least to give them the comfort of knowing there are plenty of others in the same boat. People should never have to feel alone or ashamed for simply being open and honest about who they are and living their truth. A family should not have to move to live in peace when others are ignorant and just plain rude. Even in families where everyone is comfortable with their gay relatives and it's all considered very normal, kids are still going to be exposed to environments where it isn't. It's extremely important to keep the lines of communication open. Classmates can be cruel, and it is perfectly understandable if a kid who has an LGBTQ uncle, aunt, cousin, mother, or father decides to keep it a secret from even their own friends.

Perhaps if schools made more of a strategic effort to teach students how to treat people in general, and to exercise tolerance, acceptance, and patience for those who are different, then the LGBTQ community may be better understood, or those with different religious beliefs or cultures, or those with autism or other learning disabilities, or those who are overweight and so on. How can we, as a society, come together and reduce the level of cruelty going on in our schools and teach kids the simple but crucial importance of treating *everyone* with respect? How can this not be our top priority as a civilization of human beings?

A Ride with GLIDE

I interviewed Jerrell Walls, a pastor at CCOV (Christ Chapel of the Valley) in North Hollywood, California, a Christian church with predominately gay, lesbian, bisexual, and trans-gender parishioners. Jerrell worked with an organization called GLIDE (Gays and Lesbians Initiating Dialogue for Equality) in Los Angeles. GLIDE is the foremost speakers' network working to eliminate homophobia through interactive, age-appropriate presentations. They engage in dialogue with thousands of students, educators, businesses, and community groups each year, and their presentations confront the myths and stereotypes that lead to anti-LGBTQ bias, bigotry, and bullying. (For more information, go directly to their website www.socal-glide.org/.)

I went with Jerrell to a high school in Santa Monica, California, where he spoke as a representative of GLIDE to ninth- and tenth-grade students. It was very interesting to observe their perceptions about gay people. I found this group of teenagers to be a lot more informed and open-minded than when I was a teen, some twenty-odd years ago (okay, thirty-odd years ago if I'm being totally honest here).

The students were asked to share representations of LGBTQ people that they've heard or seen. This activity is a springboard for an analysis to deconstruct prejudice. I saw in the classroom that most students do not hold those beliefs themselves.

In addition to answering questions, Jerrell also asked the students many questions and he was very effective at leading the school in an informative discussion.

According to Michael from GLIDE, "We do brainstorming with the class at every engagement to create a picture of homophobia . . . before we examine those myths and stereotypes and look at their underpinnings. Following that brainstorming about what they've heard about LGBT people, each speaker tells his or her story and then there is Q&A."

The following are some questions and responses from the Q&A session with Jerrell, where Jerrell asked the students to answer some questions for him before they began their discussion:

How can you tell if someone is gay?
- "The way they act."
- "When the dude talks like a woman."
- "How they dress."
- "Neon clothes."
- "They dye their hair."
- "How they interact."
- "How they sit."
- "They're colorful."
- "A buzz cut for girls means they are lesbian."
- "By their vocabulary."
- "Sometimes you can't tell."

What causes people to be gay?
- "Media."
- "It's a choice."

- "They are born that way." (Fifteen years ago, I don't
  think "they were born that way" would have been
  an answer. Lady Gaga wasn't even around then!)

What kind of jobs do gay people have?
- "Work in a gay bar."
- "Designing clothes."
- "Hairstylist."
- "Rock bands."

What kind of jobs do lesbians have?
- "Singer."
- "Army."
- "Teacher."

What are some names gay people are called?
- "Queer."
- "Gay."
- "Fag."
- "Homo."
- "Dyke."
- "Faggot."
- "Butch."
- "Fruit."
- "Cocksucker."

These derogatory words that the kids still hear certainly are a
strong reminder of how difficult it might be for a young person
to reveal to their fellow classmates that they have a gay person in
their family or if they themselves are gay.

I am glad I was able to observe that, by the end of the class, the two men from GLIDE were able to get the students to see that many perceived ideas about LGBTQ people were unfounded, especially many of the negative stereotypes. I could tell that the stories they told moved and inspired the students and that the GLIDE men were great role models for them.

A report conducted by GLSEN titled "Strengths and Silences: The Experiences of Lesbian, Gay, Bisexual, and Transgender in Rural and Small-Town Schools," by Neil A. Palmer, MS, Joseph G. Kosciw, PhD, and Mark J. Bartkeiwicz, MS, indicated that students in rural schools more frequently experience derogatory comments than students in suburban and urban schools. Ninety-seven percent of rural LGBTQ students heard *gay* used in a negative way, such as "That's so gay." Ninety-four percent heard other homophobic language (*dyke* or *faggot*), sometimes frequently.

You Can't Show That in the Yearbook

Sometimes the problem is not the students but the school administration. For example, a photograph of student Andre Jackson kissing his boyfriend, David Escobales, been published in a New Jersey high school yearbook in 2007, but Newark school officials had decided it was inappropriate and ordered it to be blacked out of every copy of the school's yearbook. What message does censoring such a photo send to a young person who is either LGBTQ or has an LGBTQ family member?

Although that particular photo controversy occurred back in 2007, there are certainly many high schools that would make the same decision today. However, more recent incidents suggest that the tide is definitely turning. In 2013, a photo of a homosexual couple won "cutest couple" at a New York high school, beating out all the heterosexual couples who entered their photos. A student from that high school posted the image from the yearbook onto her Tumblr and, according to the *Huffington Post*, it was shared nearly 100,000 times within the first twenty-four hours. An even more recent event occurred at a Washington high school in 2015. A transgender student was voted homecoming queen by her graduating class at Renton High School and the touching story not only went viral in social media but was covered by major news outlets as well.

Sometimes the problem is more with the teachers than with the students or school administrators. Take, for example, a New Jersey teacher who wrote a Facebook post in 2012 about how she found same-sex relationships immoral. While every US citizen is entitled to free speech, we must consider that this came from a teacher who was supposed to be objective about her students and not voice her strong opinion in a place where her students would surely be able to see it. Not only did this woman make her personal bias against LGBTQ people very clear, but her message could be taken as a call to action for everyone else to take a stand against the LGBTQ community, as well.

Further south, as of 2013, more than a hundred schools in the state of Georgia said "No Gays Allowed!" Georgia lawmakers wanted to take this even further and add millions more to the $170 million program already in place to support schools that explicitly ban gay and lesbian students.

Another recent case in Ohio reveals how nontolerance can also be applied to teachers. Carla Hale, a teacher in Clintonville, Ohio, was fired just days after an anonymous parent informed the school that Carla's partner's name had appeared in her mother's obituary. Carla had been a teacher at the school for nineteen years, and instead of showing her any sympathy about her mother's passing, they terminated her employment within the same week.

Documentaries That Schools Should Show

Lesléa Newman, the author of *Heather Has Two Mommies*, told me about a must-see documentary, *It's Elementary: Talking About Gay Issues in School*. It was produced by Helen Cohen and Debra Chasnoff, an Academy Award–winning documentary filmmaker who also directed the film. Sadly, Debra passed away in November 2017.

The groundbreaking film came out in 1996 and was one of the first to show how antigay prejudice affects children. The documentary provides adults with practical lessons on how to talk to children about LGBTQ people, and also looks at family diversity from a kid's point of view. I feel it is something that should be made available in every school library.

In 2007, Chasnoff directed a sequel titled *It's STILL Elementary* to look back on why *It's Elementary* was originally produced, the response it got from the conservative right, and how it helped the national "safe schools" movement. Some of the original students who appeared in the documentary film were in the sequel, as well. Most importantly, the film showed that children are eager and willing to think about stereotypes and learn new facts about what it means to be gay or lesbian.

It's Elementary was shot in six schools, both public and private, and it provides a clear picture of what happens when kids from kindergarten through eighth grade talk about LGBTQ related topics in age-appropriate ways. It showed excellent teaching about family diversity, name-calling, stereotypes, community building, and more.

Despite its success, the film has been relentlessly condemned by the conservative right. Perhaps one reason is that the film also showed footage of a legislator trying to stop LGBTQ subjects being taught in schools, saying, "We can and we must protect the taxpayers by keeping this trash out of our schools. And that's exactly what it is. It's trash." For anyone who would like to decide for themselves, *It's Elementary* is available through the GroundSpark website (www.groundspark.org). I personally thought it was excellent and particularly enjoyed the students in the film addressing the class speakers with some very interesting questions and comments:

"I heard gay men keep their houses clean."

"How do you find out if the other person is gay or lesbian?"

"How do your parents feel about you being gay?"

"Did anyone tell you they don't want to be your friend anymore when you told them you were gay?"

"Is there a reason why you are gay? Were you raped or did you go through something?"

"If you have kids, how old would you want them to be before you tell them?"

"If you had a choice to like start all over and be straight, would you rather be straight?"

"If you had kids who said they want to be gay like you, what would you say?"

"Do you get upset when people call you names?"

During the documentary, they also spoke with fourth graders, and one of the girls said, "The adults say it's wrong to be gay, you shouldn't do it. I think it's just the way a person is, you can't change it." And a boy in the class said, "So what if someone is gay, like what's the big whoop?"

In the film, a teacher tells the class about famous gay people and played the song "Circle of Life" from the film and Broadway show *The Lion King*. He then asked who the singer was and one kid answered, "The Lion King." Then someone else said, "Elton John," and the look on the face of one of the girls when she heard that Elton John was gay is priceless. This same girl made this very important observation years later when interviewed for *It's Still Elementary*: "Education is never wrong if you present the facts."

That last sentence should be said to those still opposed to bringing this subject into schools, such as the religious groups who also opposed the film, saying, "It was a very calculated attempt by gay activists to recruit the next generation of sex partners."

A different class in the film was asked to think of words that first came to mind about gay people. Some of the words were *happy, hug, pair, unrealistic, couple, sick, gross, cross-dressing, sex, man, woman, kissing, weird,* and *twenty-five cents.* (That last one was my favorite answer, and made me wonder where that kid had been hanging out.)

While the film certainly had some good moments of humor, the questions and comments that came from a few of those kids truly revealed how much misinformation they can be exposed to either from what they hear on TV, from their fellow students, or even their own family. Not only did the film portray just how important it is for this subject to be discussed in school, but it also showed how important it is for teachers to step in when kids are saying derogatory things or taunting other students.

Otherwise, kids will take the teacher's tolerance of bad behavior as further reinforcement that there is something wrong with LGBTQ people, which can be especially harmful to those who are LGBTQ or know someone who is.

The sequel, *It's Still Elementary*, is also available from the GroundSpark website, and I highly recommend it, too. A child from the original 1996 documentary was interviewed in the sequel and revealed his older perspective: "The documentary made me realize to accept people for who they are rather than based on their personal life. If they don't do anything to harm you, then there's no reason to be mean to that person."

A girl from the original film who also appeared in the sequel said, "It gave us a forum to ask questions we wanted to ask." Adults who saw the original documentary were also asked to give their thoughts on the sequel, and many of them expressed how wholesome and innocent the discussions were.

According to one of the boys who was in the original film, it was a tremendous relief. "The day they filmed my classroom for the film, a burden was lifted from my shoulders, because I realized I might be gay."

Debra Chasnoff: Director of Several Helpful Documentaries Shown In Schools

I had a chance to interview Debra Chasnoff, a couple of years before she passed, to get the director's perspective of these films. She explained that she was inspired to do *It's Elementary* because she was a lesbian parent and was concerned about what her son, who was five at the time, would encounter when he started school. She wanted to do a project that would address safety from antigay harassment and would discuss what to do or say when kids ask, "Why are they saying bad things about the people I love the most?"

Debra had already won an Oscar for her documentary *Deadly Deception—General Electric, Nuclear Weapons and Our Environment*, and she was the first lesbian to thank her partner in her acceptance speech for the award.

Debra decided to combine her knowledge and skill of documentary filmmaking and her passion for social change. In 1980, she and Kim Klausner took over Women's Educational Media, founded by Liz Dimond. Debra became the director and has been in the leadership position since then. In 2007, it was renamed GroundSpark. For LGBTQ families who specifically need help in discussing the topic with children, Debra also made another film called *That's A Family!*, which is available on Amazon.com or directly from the GroundSpark website. She said, "For parents that are nervous about talking with kids about gay people, the film can do the talking, or at least start the conversation and allow parents to ask the kids what they thought about someone having a gay parent, or kids having two moms, etc."

Although Debra's films are now shown in quite a few schools and there have been many changes toward a more accepting view of LGBTQ people, she had said that many schools were still reluctant to allow this subject to be taught or even discussed, as some people claim this kind of teaching in schools, or showing same-sex parents raising kids, has a negative impact on the students. However, Debra also felt that this attitude is about to change quite dramatically as more people are beginning to realize the opposite. "*Not* showing it would have a negative impact on the kids. By seeing and learning, they become more open-minded and supportive of people who are different."

A Guide for Teachers and LGBTQ Parents

The Family Equality Council has a booklet called *Opening Doors*, which is an excellent guide for teachers and LGBTQ parents. It discusses many of the fears everyone has:

Children may fear that their families will be called names and not be included in certain school activities, friends might not be allowed over for sleepovers, and teachers and kids may assume they are LGBTQ.

LGBTQ parents may fear that their child may be discriminated against or not invited over to other families' houses, that the school may out them and they will risk losing their jobs, that their family won't be reflected in the curriculum.

Teachers or schools may fear that they will have to talk about sex in the classroom, and that if they are inclusive, they could be accused of promoting homosexuality.

The larger school community may fear that their children will be influenced to be gay and the traditional family will be devalued.

The booklet also discusses how silence can be just as powerful as the spoken word, if not more so. When children do not feel welcome to talk about their families at school, they are forced to leave a significant part of their lives behind when they enter a school or childcare setting. This can also have a negative impact on their

(continued)

self-esteem. When children do not feel comfortable in a school environment, their learning and development can be negatively affected as well.

Also interesting is what their findings reveal about children with one or more LGBTQ parents. Most of these children do not view their families as different or deficient. For these children, like all children, their families are just their families. However, children encounter negative messages about LGBTQ people in the world outside of their homes, and as a result are made painfully aware of the differences and the possible physical, social, and emotional dangers of disclosing that they have one or more LGBTQ parents. Because they are sensitive to—and fearful of—the repercussions, children may choose to never talk about their families within the school community. The booklet stresses that adults need to respect these feelings, providing advice to parents and teachers with regard to schools, including encouraging schools to have teachers use inclusive language for all families, especially theirs, especially in awkward situations like Mother's Day or Father's Day, and to find a way to contribute to your school's community, like PTA meetings and classroom trips. Educators must make sure all students feel safe at school, stop harassment and bullying comments, and let them know that certain hurtful words will not be tolerated.

Not only is it important that children know about their LGBTQ relatives, but all students must learn to be supportive of LGBTQ students and students with

LGBTQ family members. The more kids who know people who are LGBTQ or know kids whose relatives are LGBTQ, the less kids will participate in the name-calling and bullying of LGBTQ classmates and LGBTQ people, and the less kids will be willing to tolerate those who do. Perhaps soon it will be the reverse situation, where students worry more about being "outed" as bullies because everyone knows how "totally uncool" it is to be cruel.

CHAPTER 7

Religion:
Pray the Gay Bashers Away

Religion, or rather the way it's perceived by some, can be divisive and sometimes spreads hate toward LGBTQ people, which is one of the biggest issues they have faced. I came across this a lot in my interviews and I see it a lot on social media as well.

Religions may disagree on many things, but their most conservative adherents all seem to unite in their belief that being gay is evil and a sin. For instance, Islam, Christianity, Mormonism, and Judaism (or at least the way some interpret these religions) all believe homosexuality is not just a sin but an abomination. Judaism believes "it is not kosher," but it does appear that many modern Jewish people are okay with it.

I was not raised in any particular religion, but my mother is Protestant and my father came from a Muslim family, although he didn't practice it himself. I do remember my Turkish grandmother prayed five times a day. My parents decided not to bring us up with any religion and let us decide for ourselves if we wanted to practice one. My mother did teach us the bedtime prayer, "Now I lay me down to sleep, I pray the Lord my soul to keep," and we said grace sometimes before meals: "God is great, God is good, now let's thank Him for our food." Like many families we knew, we celebrated Christmas and Easter. I guess my mom did sneak in a little religion in raising us, but in order to write this book I needed to go outside my family to find out how different religions viewed homosexuality, and I will be discussing what I found in this chapter.

Some people, including family members, use religion to attack or make LGBTQ people feel as if they are not as worthy. Children and adults may be hearing antigay attitudes in the "name of God." While bigots exist in all faiths, there are also safe spaces for religious members of the LGBTQ community, and there are many good religious leaders. I'll start by breaking down what some of the major religions feel about homosexuality and then I'll briefly touch on a few bad eggs to highlight what we continue to deal with and the problems they create before moving quickly to the good ones with stories and solutions.

World Religions

Christianity

According to a 2014 study by the Pew Research Center, 70.6 percent of the adult population in the United States identified themselves as Christians, and there are many denominations in Christianity. We also tend to see more on TV and social media here in America related to Christianity, so I may have used a few more examples in this chapter about that particular religion. However, all religions, in my opinion, are equally important, but I will start with what Christianity has to say about homosexuality.

The many Christian denominations vary in their positions, from condemning homosexual acts as sinful, through being divided on the issue, to seeing it as morally acceptable. Even within a denomination, individuals and groups may hold different views. Further, not all members of a denomination necessarily support their church's views on homosexuality. For example, the Roman Catholic Church views as sinful any sexual act not related to procreation by a couple joined under the Sacrament of Matrimony. The Church considers "homosexual acts" to be "grave sins" among other things and "under no circumstances can they be approved." All Orthodox Church jurisdictions, however, welcome people with "homosexual feelings and emotions" while encouraging them to work toward "overcoming its harmful effects in their lives" and not allowing the sacraments to people who seek to justify homosexual activity. The Catholic Church requires those who are attracted to people of the same (or opposite sex) sex to practice chastity, because it teaches that sexuality should only be practiced within marriage, which includes chaste sex as permanent, procreative, heterosexual, and monogamous.

There are a few more denominations with similar beliefs, many against homosexuals, however I've noticed many churches in most of the denominations are becoming more accepting of homosexual relations and welcoming of LGBTQ individuals and families.

Mormonism

In 2013, the Mormon Church launched a new website, Mormonsandgays.org, to establish its official stance on homosexuality, saying that gay people were born this way. As recently as 2008, however, Mormons didn't accept "biological determination for same-sex attraction."

Interestingly enough, the church has changed its position, stating, "Individuals do not choose to have such attractions." The website features numerous videos of church leaders speaking about AIDS counseling and urging parents not to reject their children who "pursue a gay lifestyle."

Aside from aiming to clarify the church's standing on homosexuality, the website also follows up by promoting a message of extending love and understanding to gay people and "responding sensitively and thoughtfully" when encountering those with same-sex attraction. However, the church also makes it clear that its "tolerance" is far from acceptance. "That we cannot do, for God's law is not ours to change." Therefore, there is no changing the church's position of what is morally right. The Book of Mormon actually makes no references to homosexuality, but the church maintains that while "the attraction itself is not a sin, acting on it is." When you really think about it, Mormonism still isn't all that different from the views of other religions, such as Catholicism—only instead of just asking gay followers to abstain from gay sex, Mormonism actively seeks to "pray the gay away" with counseling. It aims to train gay people to be able to exist in heterosexual marriages, since marriage is a very important tenet of the religion. Videos of some of these "success" stories are also available on the site. Most, if not all, gay people will tell you that you simply cannot pray the gay away.

Islam

The following is from IslamOnline.net and was written by the website's health and science editor, Dr. Nadia El-Awady. She addressed the subject to the one-seventh of the world's population that follows the Muslim religion.

Al-Qaradawi states that Islamic beliefs are squarely against gay relationships because Allah created opposites to attract, including the attraction between man and a woman, as the means to continue the existence of the human species.

He then goes on to quote several passages from the Koran, including "For ye practise your lusts on men in preference to women: ye are indeed a people transgressing beyond bounds" (7:81). "And we rained down on them a shower (of brimstone): Then see what was the end of those who indulged in sin and crime!" (7:84).

These passages refer to the People of Lut in the Koran, whose behavior, and the condemnation of God upon it, are remarkably similar to Sodom and Gomorrah in the biblical book of Genesis. There are gay Muslim groups just as adamant as their Christian and Jewish counterparts in declaring that their holy scriptures and religious philosophy do not oppose homosexuality. I researched and found mosques that are gay and lesbian friendly and believe in gender equality, with mixed gender prayers led by a woman, many of which are part of the Members of Muslims for Progressive Values network of mosques.

Judaism

The Torah forbids the homosexual act known as *mishkav zakhar*, but it says nothing about whether homosexuality is a state of being or a personal inclination. In other words, according to traditional Judaism, a person with a homosexual inclination can be an entirely observant Jew, as long as he or she does not act out that inclination. The subject of homosexuality in Judaism dates back to the Torah, in the books of Bereshit and Vayiqra. Bereshit (Genesis) discusses the destruction of the cities of Sodom and Gomorrah by God. Vayiqra (Leviticus) forbids sexual intercourse between males, classifying it as a *to'evah* (something abhorred or detested), which can be subject to capital punishment under "halakha" (Jewish law).

The basis of the prohibition against homosexual acts derives from two biblical verses in the Old Testament and in Leviticus: "Do not lie with a male as one lies with a woman; it is an abhorrence" (Leviticus 18:22) and "If a man lies with a male as one lies with a woman, the two of them have done an abhorrent thing; they shall be put to death—their bloodguilt is upon them" (Leviticus 20:13). The Torah also considers a homosexual act between two men to be an abhorrent thing (*to'evah*), punishable by death—a strong prohibition.

I was told to watch the documentary *Trembling Before G-d* to get a much better understanding of homosexuality and Judaism. It was directed by Sandi Simcha Dubowski and gives an interesting and accurate portrayal of various gay Orthodox Jews who struggle to reconcile their faith and their sexual orientation. It showed how common it is for family members to be disowned simply because of religious beliefs and how many rabbis (just like priests and pastors) just can't accept that it is okay to be gay. They believe that if someone does happen to have those feelings, they must suppress them, as acting on them is an act against their faith. The documentary portrayed a teenager who told his rabbi he thought he was gay. The rabbi told the boy it was an abomination and made him go to a psychiatrist. Twenty years later he went back to visit the rabbi and let him know that it wasn't possible to change his sexuality. He also wanted to know if the rabbi still had the same beliefs as he did twenty years ago. Unfortunately, nothing had changed with the rabbi and although he seemed genuine in wanting to help, he represented the religious leaders who continue to do more harm to gay people than good. Oy vey.

I was curious to see if there were any gay/lesbian synagogues and was surprised to find quite a few. One is called the BCC (Beth Chayim Chadashim), located in Los Angeles, California, and is described as a progressive and diverse community of people who come together to celebrate Jewish faith and culture. Established in 1972, it was the world's first synagogue founded by, and with an outreach to, lesbians and gay men. The current leader, Rabbi Lisa Edwards, is a lesbian married to Tracy Moore, and while the BCC sustains a Jewish community for gay, lesbian, bisexual, and transgender Jews, they welcome all who wish to join the community with them. I also found Congregation Beth Simchat Torah in New York for LGBTQ Jews. CBST offers a spiritual home in the city and since it was founded in 1973, it has grown to 850 members, making it the largest Jewish LGBTQ congregation in the world.

Buddhism (Pray It Forward)

Personally, I'd rather listen to Dolly Parton than the Dalai Lama, but I do have respect for him. I found out he represents only 3 to 4 percent of Buddhists. I also found out that there are several different types of Buddhists. Nevertheless, I was curious about his take on homosexuals, and it didn't take long to figure that out. Apparently, he attended a conference and met with members of the San Francisco gay community in 1998 to discuss the Tibetan Buddhist proscriptions against gay sex. During the meeting, he basically reiterated the traditional view that gay sex was sexual misconduct. This view was based on restrictions found in Tibetan texts that he could not, or rather would not, change. But there are many Western dharma communities known for their tolerance, and the Dalai Lama himself has even had openly gay students. It's rare to hear of anyone being drummed out of a Western Buddhist community for being gay, and in almost all Buddhist traditions practiced in the West—including the Tibetan communities—sexuality is rarely, if ever, an issue.

Major Players

Antigay Rhetoric from a Religious Leader Brought into Your Living Room

I was flipping through the channels (we guys love the remote control regardless of orientation) on June 9 (my birthday), 2009, and I came upon *The 700 Club* with televangelist Pat Robertson. In this particular episode, a mother had emailed Pat, saying that she was confused and didn't know how to handle the news that her teenage son had told her he was gay. He told her to tell him that being gay is an abomination and that he was going to hell.

During another episode on July 8, 2013, Pat Robertson was commenting on pictures of same-sex couples on Facebook and then went on to cite a biblical passage from the Old Testament that basically calls for the death of homosexuals. This man is given a platform on TV and, if kids see this, they are being told their LGBTQ family member is going to hell. The simplest advice here may be not to seek advice from some televangelists and clergy.

Pastors Who Should Be Put Out to Pasture

On November 30, 2013, Pastor Steven Anderson of Faithful Word Baptist Church in Arizona passionately declared that no "queers" or "homos" were allowed in the church, and never will be as long as he was pastor. "If you executed the homos like God recommends you wouldn't have all this AIDS running rampant." Children are subjected to these messages. And, often, their parents reinforce these beliefs as facts.

Then there are pastors like Kevin Swanson, who blamed Colorado wildfires on a kiss between State House Majority Leader Mark Ferrandino and his partner. Pastor Swanson is also blaming the gay kiss for the recent floods that hit the state—which, wow, that must have been one wet kiss to cause all that flooding.

Then there is Pastor Charles L. Worley of Providence Road Baptist Church in Maiden, North Carolina, whose "solution" to the so-called gay scourge was to trap queers and homosexuals behind an electric fence so they can't get out.

Another "man of the cloth" who used his job to spread bigotry and hatred was Fred Phelps. He founded the Westboro Baptist Church in 1955. Though he died in 2014, the Topeka-based group he founded has continued their vehement antigay rhetoric and picketing of funerals with signs saying things like "God Hates Fags."

I did not write this book to bash Christianity; my purpose is to bring awareness to the fact that many religious leaders are spreading antigay rhetoric that is not only untrue but also harmful for children to hear. In fact, religion is among the biggest issues for families of LGBTQ people. There are religious leaders that don't even follow what Jesus taught. They preach incorrect things that kids with LGBTQ family members may ultimately hear. They are essentially leading these kids to believe that they and their family are worth less than other families. They are being told to condemn people in their family who have not done anything wrong; they just happen to be gay. That can do so much damage to a young mind.

Sometimes the words of these people can sting but I remember as a kid learning that if you ignore a bee, it will go away. Not sure if that's true but maybe that is a solution? Tell kids to ignore these "bees" and this kind of talk (buzz). Let kids know there is a lot of disinformation on TV and not everything they see on TV is true (some adults need to learn this too) and be ready to debunk it. Let them know some people just don't know any better. Maybe tell them God loves everyone.

Religious Leaders Who Spread Love

Not all religious leaders or religious people think and act this way. In fact, many are helping to do a lot more good. Things have been changing even more since Pope Francis became the head of the Catholic Church in 2013. He is by far the most progressive pope in the history of the Church, and he proved this in his response to a reporter's question about gay priests. "If someone is gay and he searches for the Lord and has good will, who am I to judge?" Many believe that Pope Francis's statement was a powerful stand that could ultimately save lives. Think about the solace of those words to the many religious LGBTQ teenagers who have contemplated suicide because they've been told how evil they are in the eyes of their god.

Pope Francis has continued to make headlines for statements that preach tolerance and acceptance of LGBTQ people. In September 2014, he said in a highly publicized interview that the Church shouldn't interfere spiritually with the lives of LGBTQ people. He also said the Church cannot focus solely on opposing abortion, contraception, and marriage equality. Although there has been no change in official Catholic doctrine that condemns homosexual acts and opposes marriage equality, the pope's influence has proven to be more powerful than the written word. In 1992, Sinéad O'Connor ripped up a picture of then Pope John Paul II during her televised appearance on *Saturday Night Live*. She did it to spark a public protest of some of the pope's conservative teachings. I can't help but wonder: Would she praise the pope today?

Another religious leader who teaches love is Dan Birchfield of Westminster Presbyterian Church. He spoke at the funeral of Lawrence King, a fifteen-year-old who was killed because he was gay. As Reverend Birchfield stood in front of a large photograph of the victim, he said, "God knit Larry together and made him wonderfully complex." The reverend told the crowd, "Larry was a masterpiece."

Pastor Jerrell Walls: Putting Into Perspective the Passages About Homosexuality

I spoke at length with Pastor Jerrell Walls at CCOV (Christ Chapel of the Valley). He is an openly gay pastor at the independent Christian church in North Hollywood, California, where "*Everyone* is accepted." The church attracts hundreds of people to its weekly services. Pastor Jerrell and I had an in-depth discussion about the whole concept of being gay and being a Christian. He revealed something very interesting: he had come to realize the passages were not saying what we always thought they said. "Jesus never says a word about being gay, and there are only six passages that people pull out of the Old Testament that say anything about homosexuality," Pastor Jerrell said. The Old and New Testaments also say no tattoos, no pork, no mixed clothing, and that you can sell children into slavery. Obviously, most people don't follow many of these passages, so certainly the passages about homosexuality can be up for question as well. The scripture teaches us that everyone should be accepted and that God's grace covers all our sins.

I listened to an interview Pastor Jerrell did on a show called *The Nakid Truth* (the show spells it this way) on YouTube; they were discussing religious passages about being gay. While Jerrell didn't seem to change the radio host's opinion about God being against homosexuals, he did make some excellent points during the show. One thing he said to the host really hit the mark: "Maybe we need to quit going by what tradition of man has taught us and look at what was God really saying. The purpose of Christ is to draw all people to Himself. Scripture should never be used to cast people out."

Pastor Rob Bell: Supporting Marriage Equality

A very popular evangelical megachurch pastor, author, and television writer, Pastor Holmes "Rob" Bell Jr. recently went public with his support of marriage equality. Bell founded the Mars Hill Bible Church in Grandville, Michigan, which has become one of the fastest-growing churches in America. In 2011, *Time* magazine named Bell to its list of the 100 Most Influential People in the World. In 2012, he resigned as pastor of the Mars Hill Bible Church to continue his work elsewhere. He told the *Huffington Post*, "I am for marriage. I am for fidelity. I am for love, whether it's a man and woman, a woman and a woman, a man and a man." Bell went on to say, "We have supported policies and ways of viewing the world that are actually destructive. And we've done it in the name of God and we need to repent."

Too bad some of the other modern evangelists don't share this view. For example, Joel Osteen, who seems to have old-fashioned views on homosexuals. In an interview with Soledad O'Brien on CNN on September 20, 2012, Osteen said, "Being gay is a sin and gay people are not God's best work." Well, bless his little heart.

What these examples show is that religious leaders who are true leaders and not afraid to take a stand for their personal beliefs and stand up for others are getting much more recognition than those who continue to spread hate.

Here's to You, Mr. Robinson: First Priest In An Openly Gay Relationship

Vicky Gene Robinson is another religious leader who is helping to change views on homosexuality. He is from Fayette County, Kentucky, and is a retired bishop of the Diocese of New Hampshire in the Episcopal Church. He is also the first priest in an openly gay relationship to be consecrated as a bishop in a major Christian denomination believing in the historic episcopate.

I watched his documentary, *Love Free or Die*, which showed how Robinson was conflicted in his love for God and his love for his partner, Mark. He inspired many people as he traveled all over and spoke in small-town churches, Washington's Lincoln Memorial, and London's Lambeth Palace, asking bishops, priests, and ordinary people to stand up for equality.

Rev. Dr. Sean B. Murray: Churches Accepting Of All People

I contacted my mother's former pastor, Rev. Dr. Sean B. Murray, to get his insight on the subject. I had always found him to be a very nice man and I attended a few of his sermons in Syosset, New York, over the years when I was visiting my hometown. He also officiated at the wedding of my brother and his wife. After more than twelve years as pastor at the Community Church of Syosset, Rev. Dr. Sean B. Murray transferred to the First Congregational Church of Riverhead, whose mission statement states:

> "We are an open and affirming congregation in which all persons regardless of race, ethnic background, economic status, gender, age, personal ability, or sexual orientation, are equally affirmed into membership, leadership and employment, and are joyfully welcomed."

Pastor Murray holds a master of divinity degree from Union Theological Seminary and a doctorate from the New York Theological Seminary. But aside from his credentials, Pastor Murray has always impressed me with his humble and grateful attitude. "I have been very lucky for all these years to have been involved with people and churches in the New York/Long Island area that are very accepting of all people, even back in the 1980s," he said during our discussion. "In New York and Long Island, quite a few very conservative areas still exist. Some of those churches are somewhat antigay, but God bless the churches that teach that the radical are welcome."

He also revealed something I found very interesting. "There are some same-sex couples that attend this church, and most of the kids there know they are couples. So it is a normal thing for them," he said. I asked about what happens when the kids hear some politician or religious leader condemn gay people and how to handle that. He responded, "We can't control the noise and crap outside of our homes, or outside our environment where there is prejudice, but we can make our environment one of genuine love and embracing of all, so the children can know those are safe places to talk about it, or where they can go for comfort."

Pastor Murray gave his honest conclusion about the continuing controversy: "They sometimes lose some members of a church when an openly gay pastor is brought in. For some older people who are from a generation where they were taught that gay was wrong or a psychological disorder, it was hard to change those beliefs, but younger people are just more accepting." That statement is exactly what I have continually discovered throughout my research for this book.

Keeping the Faith and Being Proud of a Gay Son

I attended a PFLAG meeting featuring guest speaker Wendy Williams Montgomery, who is Mormon. At the request of the church, she had participated in helping to get Proposition 8 passed, a California bill that prevented same-sex marriage. Ironically, she later found out her thirteen-year-old son was gay.

She became torn between her faith and her family, but in the end she said that she always knew her family was more important. She began educating herself and reading as much as she could on the subject of homosexuality. At the meeting, she told us that a blog written by Mitch Mane, an openly gay Latter-Day Saint, really helped her (http://www.mitchmayne.com).

Admirably, Wendy did not do what many Mormon parents do, which is kick their child out of the home for being gay. Unfortunately, many church members turned their back on the family, and Wendy's relationships with her own siblings were shattered. Wendy also knew that when she and her son went to their first PFLAG meeting, they would be entering the lion's den. She immediately acknowledged to the group that she helped take away their rights through her support of Prop 8, and for that she was very sorry. She explained that she just didn't know the damage that the law caused and how hurtful it was to people with LGBTQ families.

At the time of our conversation, Wendy and her family still went to the same Mormon church, despite the fact that many of their old friends no longer spoke to them and they didn't really feel welcome there. (Later, she and her family moved to Arizona.) She said that they are proud of their son but they also still believe in their faith, and they go to church to help dispel ignorant ideas of what it is to be gay so that other members who are gay can be more open. She said that they didn't want to leave their church at first, partly because there were so many things about it she loved, but mostly because "If you leave, you lose your voice in making a difference." Wendy also explained that she wanted to stay for others who may be there and afraid to come out. She stayed so at least one friend was sitting with that person. But it certainly wasn't easy for the family to continue attending. Wendy's son even said, "It is so hard to find Christ in this church." Nevertheless, Wendy's advice to other Mormon parents of gay kids was to do what she did: go to online support groups to read and educate yourself.

Her husband, Tom Montgomery, spoke at the meeting as well, and advised the audience on how to speak to religious people who are antigay. He said it won't work if you try to break down or attack their faith; their defenses go up and they stop listening. (This goes for all LGBTQ members and all religions.) Instead, he said to focus on the fact that if you reject your child, there are consequences. He said to stress the importance of what is going to be best for their loved one, and to warn them that children who are rejected by their parents or church are eight times more likely to commit suicide (in fact, the highest suicide rate in the United States is among gay Mormon teens). There is also a higher risk of rejected gay teens participating in risky behavior or drug use. Tom's advice was that if you come from this angle, and if you realize their beliefs come from the culture they were raised in, you may actually gain allies, one by one.

At the meeting, Wendy mentioned a time that she was speaking to another audience about her experience of being Mormon and having a gay son. Afterward, a teenage boy who was a total stranger came up to her and hugged her tightly for a very long time without saying a word, and then he walked away. She assumed he was probably gay and perhaps rejected by his own parents. She said moments like that help her know she is doing the right thing by speaking out. She said, "I am a better person for having a gay son. I judge less and love more. I have been on both sides of this issue and this is the right side, the side of truth, love, and compassion." She recommended every-one read a book that helped her deal with the issue, called *No More Goodbyes: Circling the Wagons around Our Gay Loved Ones* by Carol Lynn Pearson. The author is a Mormon who had learned her husband was gay.

The Montgomery family is also part of the Family Acceptance Project, which is a research, intervention, education, and policy initiative at San Francisco State University. It works to prevent health and mental health risks for LGBTQ children and youth, including suicide, homelessness, and HIV in the context of their families. The organization makes movies about faiths and ethnic groups, including one about the Montgomerys called *Families Are Forever*. The website is http://familyproject.sfsu.edu/.

Is That a Bible in Your Pocket or Are You Just Unhappy to See Me?

In the Bible, Jesus curses a fig tree for being barren, leading some to believe he disliked figs or fruits. I saw an amusing post on Facebook that addresses those "Jesus Hates Fags" signs. It showed a picture of Jesus with his hand over his head and the meme said: OMFG YOU GUYS . . . I SAID I HATE "FIGS."

Some may think that post is blasphemous, but I prefer to believe that God has a sense of humor and that he prefers to love and laugh with all of us, rather than "hate" some of us.

Questions and Answers about Religion

I asked people the following question on a survey during the course of my research. Here are a few of the responses.

Has religion played a part in or affected your family?

- **John:** My husband and I are atheists (both originally Catholic). Our son's teacher told us that one day at school, a girl was talking about God and angels being all around her. My son challenged her: "How do you know they're there or real?" This teacher asked my son about our family's religion. His answer was: "Daddy D. No god. Daddy S. No god. Me . . . I'm only six and I'll make up my mind later." It was the perfect answer.

- **Allison:** Yes. Our girls attend preschool at the local Jewish Community Center, though we are not Jewish. The school celebrates Jewish holidays and stories, so there's a fair amount of stuff about God. Luckily, nothing about gay people. The school is very gay-friendly, with at least three other gay-parent families there. Having the girls there has led us to talk more about religion versus atheism, the difference between stories and history, and in general our own beliefs about religion.

- **James:** Yes, we have tried to find a friendly church, which has been hard to find.

- **Jason:** Yes. Both myself and my partner are religious, and constantly dealt with how various denominations would accept or reject our family.

- **Suzie:** No, but our priest is openly gay, so not an issue.

Stuart Bell and the Prayer Warriors

Stuart Bell is the CEO and owner of Growing Generations, the largest surrogacy agency of its kind anywhere in the world. Stuart also wrote a book called *Prayer Warriors: The True Story of a Gay Son, His Fundamentalist Christian Family, and Their Battle for His Soul*. The book is a compelling read that certainly lives up to its title. It is the true story of a gay man (Stuart) who comes out to his fundamentalist Christian family. His father organizes a brigade of "prayer warriors," a frightening tactic used by the extreme religious right against even the most loving of sons.

Although the book was published in 1999, I didn't know about it until 2013. I wanted to interview Stuart immediately after I read it. When I finally did get the opportunity to inter-view him in 2014, I was shocked when he told me that to this day, his parents still don't speak to him, nor do his two sisters. Although his brother and his wife and children are now fine with his lifestyle, they also didn't talk to him for ten years. Since they reconciled over five years ago, Stuart's twenty-five-year-old nephew has not only become totally okay with his gay uncle, the young man has a gay best friend as well. Unfortunately, it was Stuart's parents' religious beliefs that drove them to alienate their son, reject him for who he was, and pretty much destroy their family in the process. However, Stuart says that his response has been to continue showing them nothing but love, especially in the letters he sent in response to the nasty letters sent to him by prayer warriors "in the name of God." Unfortunately, his younger sisters don't speak to him—not because they don't want to, but because they don't want to go against their parents' wishes.

For those who aren't familiar with prayer warriors, it is essentially spiritual warfare against "satanic forces," according to those who use it. Some letters sent to Stuart were from people he barely knew, but his parents had asked them to write him. Stuart feels it's ridiculous how some people pick and choose which scriptures they are going to follow.

Amber Price Shared a Priceless Post

In 2012, my friend Amber Price shared this beautiful story on Facebook. With her permission, I share it here.

I want to tell you about a special family I met at an IKEA three years ago—two white women with their two little girls, both black, both shy and nervous. I said to the mothers, "How beautiful your daughters are! You just have the most gorgeous family." They smiled proudly and told me they had just brought their daughters home from Somalia, and that they were celebrating their arrival with a trip to Disneyland the next day. I asked the girls if they were excited and they both nodded their heads in a fervent "Yes!" We talked, we smiled, and as we said good-bye, I told them how blessed I felt to meet such a lovely family. I will never forget the looks on the faces of those two mothers or their "Thank you" with tears in their eyes. That's a family. And that's the kind of family I support. One that's based on love, because when it comes to family and to MY beliefs as a woman of faith, that's all that matters.

I was touched by Amber's post and included it here because she says, as a woman of faith, love is all that matters, whereas some people who claim to be of faith may look at that family differently, making claims such as "the kids should have a mother or father," or "marriage is between a man and a woman," or "God wants this or that." I agree with Amber that this family, which some people may object to, is what a family is, and love is love.

All Kinds of Love

The following is a poem I wrote that later became a song, cowritten with Paul Rolnick and played during the end credits of a film I wrote/produced called *Walk a Mile in My Pradas*.

"All Kinds of Love"
Written by Sudi (Rick) Karatas

I believe God believes in all kinds of love
We all have the right to wear a wedding band
I believe He believes in all kinds of love
I believe it's the hate He can't stand
In a world where push comes to shove
I believe, God believes, in all kinds of love
I wish all religions looked at it this way.

CHAPTER 8

Thoughts from Therapists and Psychologists

Most of the people I interviewed and surveyed for this book are everyday people relaying their personal stories. However, I also wanted to get some professional insight on the subject. I spoke to therapists and doctors on an array of topics, including how to best approach children and speak with them about LGBTQ relatives and subjects, how to handle religious objections, and divorce issues.

For the record, in 1973, the APA (American Psychiatric Association) removed homosexuality as a mental disorder from the APA's *Diagnostic and Statistical Manual of Mental Disorders (DSM-II)*.

Bill Benson, LMFT, LPCC: Using a Children's Book to Explain

Psychotherapist Bill Benson's practice, the Mental Gym, offers professional counseling, coaching, and consulting services in Los Angeles, California. Benson works with his patients to better understand and resolve problems by applying logic to emotionally driven challenges.

The Mental Gym counsels individuals, couples, and families. I interviewed Bill regarding helpful ways for parents (whether same-sex or heterosexual in orientation) to discuss same-sex partnering with their children.

Bill recommended using interactive and creative resources to assist children in formulating their own questions. Depending on the age of the child, Bill has found the picture book format useful in this process. *And Tango Makes Three,* for example, is a charming and true story about two male penguins at the Central Park Zoo who partnered and created a nest together. The story's zookeeper wanted to try an experiment, so he took an egg from another nest and gave it to the gay penguin pair. The two lovebirds took turns sitting on the egg until it hatched and then continued to care for their new baby, Tango.

Bill also suggests asking children simple, open-ended questions about the characters:

"How would you feel if you had two dads like Tango did?"

"Do you think your friends would treat you differently?"

"Do you know anyone like Tango's parents?"

Helping children work though their own questions and assumptions helps them formulate an understanding that can be gently nurtured toward compassion for others.

And Tango Makes Three was in the top five of the hundred most banned books from 2000 to 2009, according to the American Library Association, presumably because the penguins were gay. The penguin book I read as a kid, *Mr. Popper's Penguins* (later made into a movie with Jim Carrey), was not banned, maybe because all twelve penguins in that book were straight (although one out of ten people are supposedly gay, so perhaps that applies to penguins as well and one of Mr. Popper's penguins was closeted?).

Dr. David Giella: Talks Divorce Issues and Keeping It Simple

David Giella, a former casting director/producer turned psychologist, currently practicing in North Hollywood, California, pointed out that there are many complicated subjects we need to explain to kids. *What happens when someone dies? Where do babies come from?* And we also need to explain human sexuality. Dr. Giella stressed the importance of explaining such things in developmental ways that children can understand—and doing so without adults lying or sugarcoating things. For example, when explaining a gay uncle or aunt, he suggests introducing it as a simple concept based on something they already understand: "Uncle Nick loves Johnny the way Aunt Irene loves Uncle Mike."

Dr. Giella further explained, "When approaching the topic of gay people, keep it simple. Love is love. Gay is not only about sexuality. It's about relationships. When you get married, it's not about sex. You don't talk to your kids about your sex life and there's no need to tell them about their aunt or uncle's private moments in the bedroom either. It's about love, commitment, and family. You don't need to get into their sexual connection with a five-year-old. The age of the child will affect how much you need to go into detail, as there are certain concepts they don't grasp for a while until a certain age. For example, when the child is very young they can't grasp, how can *my* mommy be *your* sister?"

Dr. Giella's advice reminded me of how my father would do this with his grandkids. He would point to their mom and say, "That's my daughter!" Then one of the kids would say, "No, that's my mommy!" and back and forth they would go. The youngest child simply did not understand how his mother could also be someone's daughter. It was actually quite entertaining watching the child get so frustrated.

I also asked Dr. Giella his advice for when one parent turns out to be gay and the parents get divorced. He said, "It's not all that different from others who get divorced who are not gay. Either way, the child feels, 'You screwed up my life, everything was fine, then you did something and now it's not fine and I'm scared. I'm mad at you and it's your fault.'" Dr. Giella continued, "Don't reduce it to one aspect of being gay; it's about relationships."

When I asked for his thoughts on how to treat religion, I specifically brought up the scenario of kids who understand there is nothing wrong with having LGBTQ relatives or parents but often run into people who bring up religion, saying it's a sin and "those people" are bad. Or how kids may see some politicians and public personalities on TV saying it's wrong for gay people to marry. Dr. Giella suggested telling the kids, "Lots of people think different things. Some people who disagree with other people say really bad things about the people they disagree with and even sometimes start wars, and that's bad."

He further explained, "When talking with children, you want them to understand that people have the right to be wrong. You don't want to make it bad to be wrong. They are bad for being bad, for bad things they do, not for being wrong. If we demonize those who carry the antigay signs, then we are no better than them. We would be doing the thing we are fighting against. Don't necessarily excuse them. When talking to your child, give them a sense that the people who say bad things are wrong and it comes from lack of education. They are taught a certain thing and think that it's right. We're going to let them be wrong. A lot of people are wrong and it's okay. Holding an anti-gay sign, you're allowed. Throwing a rock and calling names, that's hurtful."

As much as I know Dr. Giella is right about just letting other people be wrong, I find it hard to do, even as an adult. Especially with those who are wrong and insist on denying other people their constitutional rights or who allow their beliefs to make them act in hateful or hurtful ways. It's hard not to get angry. However, I commend the way Dr. Giella looks at it and I believe we should all strive for his grace and maturity.

Dr. Giella also advised on how to respond if young children bring up the subject of sex. He said to give them an answer such as, "Same as men and women, they touch each other, make each other feel good, hold each other tight." It should be no different or harder to explain than a straight counterpart conversation. He also said to find out what they already know and what they think first, before you explain anything, and to arm yourself with developmentally appropriate responses and information.

Dr. Giella gave some important final thoughts: "It is true that there is a problem of possible ridicule of children by their peers as a consequence of the public recognition of the homosexual orientation of the parent. A similar problem is faced by any minority group member's child if the family resides among a largely non-minority group. Difference is not easily accepted in our culture, but it is a fact of life. Just as intelligent black or Jewish parents can help their children to cope with bigotry, so can homosexual parents."

John Dennem, MA, CADC-II, ILPCC: Transgender Thoughts, LGBTQ in the military

John Dennem is in a PhD program in Los Angeles. He grew up in a small town in Missouri with a population of three thousand, and he told me a funny story of when his sister was thirteen and one of her teachers was saying negative things about gay people at her school. She finally gave the teacher a piece of her mind, saying, "You stupid bitch, my brother is gay and he is none of those things!" Although she got suspended for lashing out, it was worth it for her to get her point across. John said, "Gay people aren't punished for being gay, so much as they are punished for telling the truth."

According to John, 84 percent of people have a family member or a friend who is gay. Many people who report they are okay with gay people still don't want to live next door to someone who is gay, though. They don't want their kids to have gay teachers and will give less effort if they have gay bosses. Interestingly enough, 54 percent of people say gays and lesbians should not be discriminated against, and many of these people support same-sex marriage. A Herek national telephone survey conducted in 2009 found that the majority of people said they had a gay friend or family member, and yet 57 percent of those surveyed said gay sex was disgusting and morally wrong.

John also had some interesting insight on the transgender community. He specifically addressed the common beliefs of religious people who say it is an abomination and God doesn't make mistakes, and that if you are born a man you should stay a man. His viewpoint and response to that line of reasoning: "Transgenderism occurs in nature. An example is the clown fish that changes sex. When the last female or male dies in the school, then one changes over to the other sex. A symbol for transgender is the butterfly. Did God make a mistake when he made the caterpillar? The caterpillar is born a caterpillar but must become a butterfly. So it is with trans persons—they must transition to become the beautiful butterfly they were meant to be all along." John also pointed out that just because a law changes doesn't mean there is immediate acceptance of such laws (i.e., marriage equality and gays in the military). He has a nineteen-year-old nephew who is currently on active duty in the marines, so he knows the Marine Corps was and remains a bastion of hypermasculinity. Although "Don't Ask Don't Tell" is supposed to be gone, machismo is still embedded in the military culture. His nephew hears many negative things about gay people and wants to say something and stand up for his uncle but feels he can't. He fears it would likely impact his career. However, John told his nephew that it is much safer for him to speak up than for the marine who is gay. His may be the voice the gay marine needs to hear to know she or he is not alone and has an ally within the platoon. John told his nephew, "Your speaking up may save that marine lots of heartache and shame."

John went on to say that society deems gay as not normal and it's something families should not be afraid to talk about. Relatives should ask the gay person, "What do you want me to know about you?" He also said, "If someone has a gay relative and someone else they know (such as another family member) says something negative about gay people, that person needs to tell other adults what they are saying is wrong. Silence is not good." Gays are the only minority that, for the most part, grow up in families that don't act or feel like them. A gay child is called "faggot," "punk," or "sissy" on the playground for the first time and they know they cannot go home and talk about it. This is because although Mom or Dad did not say anything negative about gays, the other family members who come over say negative things all the time, and Mom and Dad don't say anything to these family members when they speak negatively of the LGBTQ community. The child then gets the idea that home is not a safe place to discuss this topic for fear of being thrown away. They internalize this shame and so begins a life of struggle to compensate for shame due to heterosexism.

"Parents need to create a safe place for a child to figure things out and to let them know if they are gay. No matter who they are, they will always love them," he said.

Maurie Davidson, "Momma Mo": Unconditional Love, Consistency, Compassion, and Common Sense

Maurie Davidson, MSW, BCD, has been a clinical social worker for approximately fifty years in Southern California. She is a board member of the Los Angeles chapter of PFLAG (Parents and Friends of Lesbians and Gays) and is an adviser representing PFLAG National to the Southern California Chapter of Out &

Equal. She practices psychotherapy with individual adults, couples, families, and adolescents and specializes in relationships and life transitions. She has worked with many lesbian, gay, and bisexual adults and adolescents. Maurie is also the proud mom of a lesbian daughter and daughter-in-law, and a grandmother to their two adorable children.

She has become a good friend of mine and is known among many of her friends as Momma Mo. I asked what she saw as some advantages to having two moms or two dads, and she relayed a story she'd heard from a young woman who was a member of COLAGE. "This young lady's two dads helped her shop for clothes and makeup for her senior prom. She proudly announced she was the best looking at her prom thanks to her two gay dads. A little bit of a stereotype, as not all gay men are into fashion (myself included), but I like how she makes it such a positive thing. Another advantage is that these children are brought up by two loving people who work hard, and through extra effort bring children to love into their lives. Children of two moms and two dads also often have more of an appreciation for all kinds of families. If a woman's or man's voice is needed, this void can be filled by cultivating friendships within their own community and within the schools."

One of the biggest changes Maurie says she has noticed in the last several years is that more people now ask, "Do you have a partner or significant other?" Rather than just assuming people are always going to be with someone of the opposite sex, there seems to be more awareness of the variety of families. She also relayed a cute story about someone she knew with a young boy in nursery school. He had come home from school one day and put his hands on his hips and asked his mom, "How come I don't have two mommies?"

We also spoke of religion. "My religion is all about love, love in your heart. There's no room for negativity," Maurie said. She added, "It is important for any parent not to try to live out their dreams through their children. Power over other people has no place in raising healthy children. Children need to be raised with unconditional love, consistency, compassion, and common sense."

Dr. Davina S. Kotulski, PhD: Coming Out to Kids, Divorce Advice, and Answering Questions

Dr. Davina Kotulski is a highly-sought-after public speaker, life coach, and psychologist. She received her doctoral degree in clinical psychology from the California School of Professional Psychology and is also nationally known as a bestselling author and speaker for LGBTQ equality and self-actualization. She has written several books on marriage equality, created audio programs addressing coming out and living an authentic life, appeared in dozens of documentaries on LGBTQ equality, and been interviewed on numerous radio shows.

Dr. Kotulski has an informative audio program on her website called "How to Come Out of the Closet into Your Own Power." She says, "Anyone with a gay relative goes through their own coming-out process. They may have feelings of being separate. They may wonder, is a family member doing something bad? They may feel defensive, ashamed, or embarrassed. They may worry about what society says and what religion says. They hear things at school that may lead to a sense of confusion."

When one parent turns out to be gay and there is divorce, she suggests getting support from a professional without an expressly fundamentalist religious background or someone who attends an open and affirming church, temple, or synagogue. It should be someone who can hold the complexity of the psychological and family dynamics, knowing it's painful on both sides and that no one did anything intentionally to hurt anyone. Take into account and understand both persons' feelings. Don't side with one parent (the one that got "burned"). Be open-minded and loving. There may be blame or shame coming from the one side, such as the straight spouse wanting to blame the gay spouse for causing the problem. The straight parent should not bias the child against the gay or bisexual parent and should certainly not express hostility toward the partner in front of the child. This could be especially harmful if any of the kids turn out to be gay themselves. It could be also harmful to the child, hearing these negative things from a parent who presents themselves as being antigay.

On coming out to kids in general, Dr. Kotulski says, "It's important how we communicate when coming out. How we view ourselves. We're not a mistake. We should not be hiding or ashamed or uncomfortable. Be honest and authentic. Parents coming out should not let guilt about coming out allow children to manipulate or control you because you feel bad about coming out. Be a good parent. Set boundaries." She also mentioned the Straight Spouse Network, which supports those whose spouses are gay: http://www.straightspouse.org/.

Dr. Kotulski also suggests that parents should let their kids know about gay relatives as early as possible and in simple terms. "Girls can marry boys, some may marry girls. Some boys love girls, some boys love boys." She adds, "It's okay to show affection by holding hands or being affectionate in front of the children."

"How do two girls or two boys make a baby?" It's a question Dr. Kotulski says may likely arise, or it may come in a statement such as, "Two daddies can't make a baby." Her advice is for parents to respond using age-appropriate language such as, "Two daddies or two mommies can go to the doctor or to a special bank to get what they need to make a baby." Dr. Kotulski has also written the books *Why You Should Give a Damn About Gay Marriage* and *Love Warriors*. I personally recommend both books and her 2016 novel *Behind Barbed Eyes*. To find out more about them you can visit her website: http://www.davinakotul ski.com/.

Dr. Deborah Coolhart: Transitioning Process and Explaining to Kids

I interviewed Deborah Coolhart, who was named among the top 99 (#24) US professors in counseling, psychology, and therapy in 2013 by MasterInCounseling.org. Dr. Coolhart has been honored for her work with the transgender population as a therapist known for assisting people in the gender-transition process.

Dr. Coolhart has been teaching marriage and family therapy since 2007 at Syracuse University, where she received her MA and PhD. With her expertise in transgender familial issues, she advised, "When coming out to your children as transgender, make sure they know you are still the same person. They want to know how things are going to change, how it will affect them, and though it is a self-focused life change, you need to see the world through the kids' eyes."

She explained that the children will have concerns like: Will I be safe? How should I deal with it? Are you still my mom (or dad)? Older kids will have their own set of fears such as: What are you changing? How will that affect me? Dr. Coolhart added that the questions will vary, but the parents must be prepared to answer them.

Dr. Coolhart also explained that for trans adults, the transitioning process is extremely challenging and emotional in itself. Nevertheless, if there are kids involved, a parent still needs to be the grown-up and understand their child will likely be going through many emotions including loss, worry, concern, and embarrassment. "While it may be hurtful to you that your child is embarrassed by you, you have to be the adult," she said. She also explained that she often hears the kids saying that they feel they have to go through it by themselves and that they are forced to deal with a whole change in their family structure.

Again, Dr. Coolhart's advice for parents is to tell the kids in a way they can relate to. For example, say something like, "When I was seven, I was told I couldn't wear a certain shirt that I wanted to wear. I had to act a certain way that I didn't feel comfortable with. I was told I wasn't the right person or wasn't allowed to be the person I wanted to be. I wasn't happy for all those years. This part of me was not able to come out. But I am still the same person. Even though I wasn't happy because I couldn't truly be myself, I was happy with all the memories we have and all the things we did together, that is still the same. Like on Halloween going trick-or-treating with you, birthdays, all those memories are still the same."

Unfortunately, transgender legislation is further behind than the progress being made for gay and lesbian rights. Therefore, it is that much harder for families with transgender parents, and these parents still have to fear the possibility of losing custody of their children once they make the decision to come out.

CHAPTER 9

Celebrity Thoughts from Open LGBTQ Stars

Most people I interviewed for this book were everyday people, but I thought it would be fun to talk with just a few LGBTQ celebrities to get some of their words of wisdom and advice. I include some of their exciting accomplishments as well, so you can get to know them a little better.

Bruce Vilanch

Bruce Vilanch is one of the most talented, kindest, and most down-to-earth people in Hollywood. I had the pleasure of working with him on my film, *Walk a Mile in My Pradas*, where he played himself (brilliantly, I might add). Bruce also stars in a number of other films such as *Going Down in LA-LA Land*, *Oy Vey! My Son is Gay!*, and his documentary *Get Bruce*. However, Bruce is best known for his comedic writing of at least twenty-three Oscar telecasts, which have earned him two Primetime

Emmys and several nominations over the years. He was also head writer on the popular TV game show *Hollywood Squares*, where he sat next to Whoopi Goldberg, making us laugh. He has also written for entertainment industry icons such as Bette Midler, Cher, Donny and Marie, and *The Brady Bunch Variety Hour*. Bruce has also starred in the Broadway musical *Hairspray*.

Bruce can always be seen wearing a T-shirt with some funny saying on it, and if he isn't in the Guinness World Records for owning the most T-shirts with slogans, he soon will be. What I admire about him most is that he is a great stand-up comic and he devotes his time to doing a lot of charity and benefit performances, as well as serving on the board of the LA LGBT Center. As one of the largest gay and lesbian organizations in the world, it does a tremendous amount of work to help the LGBTQ community.

I had the privilege of sitting down with Bruce to get his perspective on the various issues addressed in this book. His first comment spoke to the main question about coming out to kids. "Attitudes have changed so much over the last several years and kids are exposed a lot more to gay figures, but it's always been about keeping it simple when explaining to kids," Bruce said. But even many years ago, or in situations where it still isn't as acceptable now, his advice would be to keep it honest and simple when explaining things to kids. "Some girls love men, some girls like girls, you'll decide later who you love," he said as an example. "The kids will have no trouble with it if you don't have trouble with it. Many times people think kids will have issues with it, when they have none at all."

Bruce then told me a good story about a woman who had her son during the hippie era and did the "hippie thing" by naming him Harmony. Years later, she regretted giving him such an odd name and started to feel guilty, realizing he might grow up being extremely bothered by his own name. She became more and more haunted and guilt-ridden, thinking that he had to go through life like that. Finally, when he was a teenager, she said to him, "You know, if you want to change your name, you can." The boy looked at her, confused, and said, "What's wrong with my name?" Yet another example of how children often don't have nearly the difficulty with things that adults assume.

Although Bruce has never had kids of his own, he explained that he is "kind of a godfather" to about forty kids. They are mostly the children of single gay parents and some lesbian couples. He explained that mothers will often establish a network of male friends as "father/male figures," so that their children can have the balance of both masculine and feminine co-parents. Bruce is often one of those guys, but he explained that he is more of an "artistic male figure" because rather than taking the kids to sports events, he'll take them to plays and musicals like *The Lion King*, which he has taken so many kids to that he has seen it about forty-five times. Bruce also joked that between him and some of the other males who co-parent, they probably add up to one full male. He pointed out that the majority of the children he knows who have been raised by gay or lesbian couples have turned out to be straight—a reality that completely contradicts the misguided people who claim kids being raised by gay people are more likely to be gay. Bruce echoed the words of many others I interviewed for this book: "The most important thing is growing up in a loving environment."

Our interview had taken place in a restaurant and during this time we both noticed two dads with a toddler at a nearby table. One of the men had been helping the little boy eat his food and he was so good with him that it was hard not to be touched. Bruce commented that when you see someone as a parent and not just as a gay person, it changes things. It adds a whole other dimension. You see them more fully and have more compassion for them as they care for their children. He added that the way Rosie O'Donnell came out, by coming out *as a parent*, was a stroke of genius.

Bruce always has words of wisdom and laughs to share and I suggest following him on Twitter to get your daily dose: https://twitter.com/thebrucevilanch.

Del Shores

I have been a fan of Del Shores ever since I saw his hilarious film *Sordid Lives*. The film features an all-star cast, including Beau Bridges, Leslie Jordan, Delta Burke, Ann Walker, Beth Grant, and Olivia Newton-John. Conceived as a "black comedy about white trash," it's one of my favorite films to this day. The sequel, *A Very Sordid Wedding*, came out in 2017 and premiered in Palm Springs as the number-one specialty box office movie in the country that week!

Del has also won many awards for writing plays and screenplays such as *Sordid Lives, Daddy's Dyin' . . . Who's Got the Will?*, and *Southern Baptist Sissies.* He also wrote several episodes of the popular TV series *Queer as Folk*, which ran on Showtime for five seasons. Del was kind enough to meet with me and discuss his experience.

I first asked him how he came out to his daughters.

"They were three and six years old when I came out. The youngest has never not known a gay dad. She doesn't remember her mom and I being together. The oldest has some memories but the majority of her memories are having a gay daddy. My ex-wife was supportive once everything was out. She was supportive of them being supportive of their dad being gay.

"I feel badly for a lot of my fans, because many times when they come out, especially in the South, they've got very evangelical ex-wives who turn the kids against them. That's such a sad thing, the kids are told that the reason your daddy left is because he is gay. So they villainize gay in that way, and then they villainize it with the Bible and the religion the gay dad once embraced.

"I remember one day I was taking the girls to school. Rebecca went to Children's Community School in the Valley, then I would drive Caroline afterward to her nursery school. On the way, Rebecca said, 'Daddy, Mommy's dating this guy named Mike, are you gonna ever date other people?' and I said, 'Actually, I've already started dating.' She said, 'You have?' I said, 'Yeah, I'm dating a guy named Simon,' and she said, 'You're dating a guy?' and I go, 'Yeah,' and she goes, 'Oh, so you're gay.' The good thing is we had gay neighbors, so she said, 'So you are gay like Dan and Ron? Oh cool.'

"I didn't expose my kids to a relationship until I thought it was indeed a relationship. The one thing that was wonderful is that Caroline and Rebecca were never ashamed of me. They were never ashamed of that part of me and they have fought for me."

I asked Del if there were any interesting things that happened at their school because they had a dad who was gay. He had quite a few stories that he shared:

"They went to Notre Dame High School in the Valley, a Catholic high school, and went to religion classes. They went to that school because of the education and the sports program. They were both softball jocks (and both straight, so there goes that stereotype). They always stood up when there were any negative things said; my little one's a real troublemaker. She was in a religion and morals class and they had to pick a controversial topic to present on. Caroline picked gay marriage and the Prop 8 issue. She made a Prop 8 video, which is on YouTube under Caroline Shores. She was so articulate at fifteen years old."

(After our interview I went online and watched Caroline's video and was very impressed.)

He told me, "Rebecca also stood up to a professor once. The professor actually said something disparaging against gays. He said, 'Gays actually harm each other.' My daughter asked if he could elaborate on that and he said, 'No, I am unable to do that in this classroom.' I guess he was saying some sort of sexual activity, so he never elaborated. She said, 'If you can't elaborate then you probably shouldn't have brought it up, and I will tell you this: I don't think my dad and my stepdad have ever harmed each other.' And then there's just like silence. I mean, like all the kids knew that her dad was gay. Afterward the professor chased her down and said, 'Rebecca, I'm really sorry if I offended you.' She said, 'Yeah, you did.' Then later Carrie had him. She's much more of a troublemaker. When she had him, he had made some comments again. Those little backhanded type of comments . . . well, those comments offended my children because their dad was gay, but there could have also been students in that class who were also gay, and hearing these comments made them feel 'less than' their straight classmates.

"One time we were at this father/daughter fund-raiser casino night at the school, we're sitting with a bunch of other parents, very liberal-minded. All these people are actors and we're sitting there playing blackjack. Caroline said, 'Daddy, my professor is coming this way, do you want to meet him?' and I said, 'Oh yeah.' As he approached she said, 'Hey, Dad, I want you to meet my religious professor I've talked to you about.' I could see he already looked nervous, so I said, 'Oh, hey, how are you?' He said 'Well, it looks like you're doing well' (referring to all the chips we had won at the gambling table), and I said, 'Yeah, gay people are good at a lot of things,' and he said, 'Well, it's good to see all of you,' and he just fled as quickly as he could."

I, of course, mentioned to Del that *Sordid Lives* is one of my favorite films and he had a cute story about that.

"When the play *Sordid Lives* came out, of course I could not show my daughters. They were too young. I would bring them in and they would watch a little bit and go out for the inappropriate parts. Then the movie came out and Carrie loved the part where Ty says, 'Momma, I'm gay.' They can quote that whole thing and they love the part where he says, 'If any more shit hits the fan.' Then all of a sudden Caroline decided she was gay, and she'd tell everybody, and very seriously she would say, 'Sharyn, I have something I need to tell you, I'm gay too.' She was seven years old at the time. She would tell everyone and get really serious and say, 'I'm also gay.' They would say, 'That's great, Caroline.' And she said, 'Daddy, I really feel we need to have a gay flag on the car.' I don't like bumper stickers but I went to West Hollywood and we put a gay flag on the car.

"Then she fell in love with this kid, this boy at school. She went to her mother and said, 'I'm so scared to tell Dad but I don't think I am really gay.' So my ex-wife calls me and tells me, 'You need to talk to Caroline because she's really concerned about telling you that she's not gay.' So I had to sit down and tell her it's okay to be straight, and she started crying and said, 'Well, I just didn't want you to be alone.' It was like the sweetest thing.

"Both of my daughters have been very active. When Prop 8 passed they went and marched with me. Carrie was so upset. 'Daddy, I've never been this upset over anything, I can't even celebrate Obama.' A couple of weeks later, she came to me and said, 'Dad, it's gonna be okay because they're all gonna die, all those haters are gonna die and my generation is gonna take care of this for you.'"

To find out more about Del and see where he is performing, check out his website: https://www.delshores.com.

Jason Stuart

Barbara Mandrell may have been "country when country wasn't cool," but Jason Stuart was openly gay when gay wasn't cool. In fact, he has been an openly gay comedian for more than twenty-five years and it certainly hasn't hurt his career yet. Besides stand-up comedy, Stuart is also well-known for his work as an actor playing both gay and straight characters on popular TV shows including *Sleepy Hollow*, *The Closer*, *Will & Grace*, *George Lopez*, *Everybody Hates Chris*, *House*, *It's Always Sunny in Philadelphia*, *Entourage*, and *Charmed*. One of his funniest roles was as Dr. Thomas, the gay family therapist on *My Wife and Kids*. In 2015, he booked a great role in *The Birth of a Nation* as a slave owner named Joseph Randall. The film set a new sales record at the Sundance Film Festival, netting a $17.5 million distribution deal from Fox Searchlight.

Jason also uses his status as an openly gay actor and comedian to support the community by performing at countless benefits supporting a variety of causes from AIDS to helping the homeless. He is the cochairman of the first-ever SAG/AFTRA LGBT Committee and also chairs the comedy shows for Lifeworks Mentoring Program.

Jason was nominated for a Gay International Film Award for best supporting actor in the independent film *Coffee Date*. He also produced and starred in his own completely improvised independent film, *10 Attitudes*, directed by Michael Gallant. He also created a very funny and moving web series called *Mentor* which he stars in with Alexandra Paul from *Baywatch* and actor/comedian Paul Elia. Of course, he also did a fantastic job playing Dr. Feist in *Walk a Mile in My Pradas*, the film I wrote and produced with Tom Archdeacon.

On the subject of religion, Jason revealed that this had been a major issue in his family. In fact, because of his sister's strong religious beliefs in Judaism, she has not allowed her children to see Jason simply because he is gay. Unfortunately, his nephews and nieces have been told by their parents what to think about gay people. Though the oldest is now in his twenties, Jason has only seen them once or twice at family funerals. It's a shame these kids have never had the opportunity to know how funny and warm their uncle Jason is. It's too bad that, because he was always open and honest about who he is, his sister kept him from knowing her children simply because of what she thinks her religion says.

However, Jason still holds the same view as many others, believing that kids should be told about their gay relatives as early as possible. "You don't need to talk about sex; it's about people who love each other and have feelings for each other and spend time together," he said. "For example, sometimes a child will walk in on their straight parents doing the 'naked pretzel' and ask, 'How come Dad was lying naked on top of Mom in bed? What were you doing?'" His advice is to answer honestly without giving any extra information. "Answer only what they ask and never make them feel they shouldn't ask questions. Just say sometimes when two people are in love they lay naked together to show their love. That's it. Later on, when they're older, you can have a more in-depth talk about the birds and the bees."

Jason's sense of humor is also seen in a comedy recording, "I'm the Daddy and I Have Candy." A mini comedy stand-up recording is available on his website: http://www.jasonstuart .com.

Chely Wright

"I am gay, and I am not seeking to be 'tolerated.' One tolerates a toothache, rush-hour traffic, an annoying neighbor with a cluttered yard. I am not a negative to be tolerated." —Chely Wright

The above quote is one of my favorites. It's from Chely Wright's compelling and candid book, *Like Me: Confessions of a Heartland Country Singer* (Random House). Chely is originally known as a country music singer/songwriter with more than twenty years of hit songs that include "Single White Female" and "Shut Up and Drive." Her first album after she came out in 2010 was called *Lifted Off the Ground*, which I can tell comes from a very personal place. Her next album, *I Am the Rain*, was released in 2016 and is one of my favorites. Chely was the first mainstream country artist to come out as a lesbian. Her moving story was chronicled in her documentary *Wish Me Away*. She has used her celebrity status to advocate for many organizations, many of which focus on helping LGBTQ youth. She is married to Lauren Blitzer and together they are raising their twin boys. Chely was kind enough to take time out of her busy schedule to speak with me by phone and share her insight.

We started off the conversation with me commenting on how far we've come and that hopefully in a few years the LGBTQ community will no longer have these issues. Chely rightfully pointed out, "Even though we have come a long way with legislation, it takes decades for hearts and minds to catch up with laws. *Loving v. Virginia* was in 1967, and today there is still much discrimination, as shown with the Trayvon Martin case and Ferguson police actions where an unarmed black man was shot and killed by police. Culture changes slower than ink and paper."

Chely also admitted that even today in New York City, where she lives, there are still certain areas where she doesn't feel comfortable holding hands with her wife. In fact, she and Lauren had an issue in a retail store on the Upper East Side where Chely said she believes a sales clerk had treated them poorly because they were lesbians. But Chely said that she contacted the CEO of the company and told him that rather than firing the employee, she preferred the store provide its workers with diversity training. Her view is that it's much better to teach and inform rather than punish. The CEO was very agreeable to her suggestion, especially since his sister is gay.

In conversation, Chely recommended the film *Small Town Gay Bar* and she said it was a story she could truly relate to her own experience growing up in a small, conservative town. She agreed that religion is one of the biggest issues that often comes up when one comes out and, unfortunately, it can create hate. In her documentary *Wish Me Away*, Chely's spiritual advisor, Rev. Dr. C. Welter Gaddy, says, "There's nobody quite as mean as people being mean for Jesus." Chely also strongly suggested watching the film *For the Bible Tells Me So* and reading the book *Crisis* by Mitchell Gold. Both deal with the topic of religion and how it affects people in the LGBTQ community.

I asked Chely if there were any affirming children's books she planned on reading to the twins when they were older (they were only sixteen months old at the time of our interview). Not surprisingly, she already had a book in mind called *Chizi's Tale*, by Jack Jones and Jacqui Taylor, which is the true story of an orphaned black rhino.

As if she weren't already busy enough, Chely also does a lot of work with organizations such as Family Equality Council, which connects, supports, and represents the over three million parents in the United States who are either lesbian, gay, bisexual, or transgender, as well as their six million children. She said, "I was very impressed with them and the tone of the event I attended. They are uniquely talking about families and rights and protections many families don't have."

Chely also founded the LIKEME Lighthouse, in 2010, which is a LGBTQ center offering an array of services for the community. Their mission is to provide a safe and welcoming space where LGBTQ individuals and their families, friends, and straight allies can come for education, resources, and to build a cohesive LGBTQ community in the Midwest. Additionally, she also serves as a board member and honorary cochair for the US organization GLSEN (Gay, Lesbian and Straight Education Network), which seeks to end discrimination, harassment, and bullying based on sexual orientation, gender identity, and gender expression in K–12 schools.

As far as speaking to kids about gay family members, Chely said there doesn't necessarily have to be a whole conversation to tell them. She also strongly believes that it will be a nonissue if parents do their job right and allow their children to be part of an environment that is fair and inclusive of all people. She explained how people should choose language that gives the message of loving everyone the same and understanding that everyone has the same liberties and rights. "Introduce the kids to Uncle Charlie and Uncle Joe. It's as simple as that," she said.

There is no better example than Chely's own nephew and niece, who were both featured in her documentary. Her eleven-year-old nephew, Max, explained how it was when he found out his aunt was a lesbian. "Her coming out made me see gay people differently. They're just like everyone else. I will admit that before I knew she was gay, I talked down about gay people. I made gay jokes. I really regret doing that." The film also shows Chely's seven-year-old niece, Amelia, reading about Chely in *People* magazine, and the conversation she had with her mom about it.

> **Amelia's mom:** "It's hard being gay . . . so what do you think?"
> **Amelia:** "It's kind of weird."
> **Amelia's mom:** "In what way?"
> **Amelia:** "Well, Dad already told me she was gay but I didn't know she was thinking of committing suicide."
> **Amelia's mom:** "Do you still love her?"

Amelia: "Yes."

Amelia's mom: "I do too. What are you going to do if anyone says anything mean?"

Amelia: "Like make fun of gay people or something?"

Amelia's mom: "Yeah."

Amelia: *"Gay people aren't bad people."*

Long before I began writing this book, I had met Chely at Fan Fair in Nashville through our mutual friend, Chuck Walter. This had been around 1997, shortly after her song "Shut Up and Drive" became a hit. She was very sweet, but I'll never forget her teasing comment about my very dark suntan at the time. "Well, you're as brown as a biscuit!" Chely's outgoing personality and open heart make her a great role model for the LGBTQ community, and I believe she got a lot of it from her father. There is a memorable clip in her documentary from when he appeared on Oprah to discuss when a child comes out to a parent. "Do not close the door, open the heart," he told the audience.

For more information on Chely, check out her website: http://chely.com/.

CHAPTER 10

Support Groups/Resources for LGBTQ Families

There are many LGBTQ groups and organizations cited throughout the book. This chapter provides a more detailed guide of my top recommended resources as well as of choices of those I interviewed.

COLAGE

COLAGE is a national movement of children, youth, and adults with one or more LGBTQ parents.

Mission: To unite people with lesbian, gay, bisexual, transgender, and/or queer parents into a network of peers, and support them as they nurture and empower each other to be skilled, self-confident, and just leaders in our collective communities.

Vision: A world in which youth with one or more lesbian, gay, bisexual, transgender, and/or queer parents are connected to a broad community of peers and mentors, are recognized as the authorities of their shared experiences, belong to respected and valued family structures, and have the tools and support to create and maintain a just society.

COLAGE seeks to build community and to progress social justice through youth empowerment, leadership development, education, and advocacy. When I started writing this book, Robin Marquis was the national program coordinator, and she was extremely helpful in providing me with lots of information about the organization and offered many suggestions on how to formulate the surveys for my research. Following her advice, I conducted several surveys online among varied demographics.

In the United States alone, more than 10 million people have one or more lesbian, gay, bisexual, transgender, and/or queer parent(s), but COLAGE is currently the only national organization in the world specifically focused on supporting children, youth, and adults with LGBTQ parents. Using their experiences and creativity, COLAGE continues to offer a diverse array of community-building opportunities, education, leadership development, and advocacy by and for kids with LGBTQ parents.

The following is taken from COLAGE materials with their permission.

What youth say about their experiences at COLAGE events:

- "COLAGE completely changed my life. It was the first time I realized that I wasn't alone and that I wasn't a freak. The classes and people I met gave me hope that I could deal with any situation and

actually enjoy the fact that my family is different."
—Ember, Arizona

- "COLAGE is important to me because everyone there is so nice and they have all helped me so much! I know it sounds corny, but I never realized how many COLAGErs there are in the world and in my area until I first was introduced to COLAGE. This is the only organization that helps children of LGBTQ families who feel like they have no one else who knows what they are going through. It also helps so many people all over the world in countless ways. Thank you to everyone at COLAGE." —Jessie, Indiana

- "When I first found out that my mom was gay I didn't really like it that much so I moved in with my dad. Then I went to COLAGE and my view on the whole thing changed. I thought it was just me, alone, but now that I have met other kids, it's easier for me." —Tom, Rhode Island

- "At COLAGE, we are all young activists by showing our pride in our families and expressing our views. Through COLAGE I became unafraid of the people who may object to what we're doing. We do all that we can to educate others about alternative families, with the hope that we will spread a spirit of tolerance and acceptance." —Morgan, California

In April 2014, I attended a COLAGE event in Los Angeles where a number of LGBTQ families led panel discussions on various issues involving the community. One of the most interesting panels was with the kids of LGBTQ parents. I thought it was also an excellent way of really helping these kids to feel included and share their experiences. They asked the kids some very introspective questions and of course there were many interesting answers. The following is from the Q&A that took place.

Has your parent coming out changed your beliefs?

- "It completely changed my worldview, made it explode into a million pieces. Nothing has ever been the same. Thank God."
- "It connected me to a larger struggle, social justice—something bigger than myself."
- "It made me realize how pointless labels are, and how we shouldn't put people in a box. Someone is not just gay or straight, they are a human being."
- "I became more open-minded and look at other people's point of view more."

Were people mean at school because of your gay parents? And how should you handle that?

- "When someone says things like 'That's so gay,' take that person aside and tell them that is not right, or that is not correct. Don't do it in front of other people."
- "Educate, don't attack the person at the moment. And ask them what are they using the word *gay* for? Why for a negative thing?"

- "Get straight friends to say something in your defense, or to tell others the phrase 'That's so gay' is unacceptable."

What do you love about COLAGE?

- "With COLAGE, you can be yourself as a person."
- "Learning from the kids."
- "Meeting new people with the same experiences."
- "Meeting someone else with the same identity, culture. So many pieces of me get to chill out."
- "We have our own experience being the children of gay parents, different than your experience. It's nice to be able to talk to people through the same lens."

Most of the kids who participated in the panel expressed feeling lucky or blessed to have a gay parent. One said, "It made my life richer and more interesting." A female participant said she was grateful for having a gay dad but only wished he had been born later because he had such a rough time back when it wasn't as acceptable.

To find out more about COLAGE, go to http://www.colage .org/ or call (855) 4-COLAGE.

PFLAG

PFLAG (Parents and Friends of Lesbians and Gays) is a national nonprofit organization with over 200,000 members and support- ers and more than 400 chapters in the United States. Founded in 1972 with the simple act of a mother publicly supporting her gay son, PFLAG is the original ally organization, now made up of parents, families, friends, and straight allies uniting with LGBTQ people. The group is committed to advancing equality through its mission of support, education, and advocacy. Their mission statement:

Our Vision: PFLAG envisions a world where diversity is celebrated and all people are respected, valued, and affirmed inclusive of their sexual orientation, gender identity, and gender expression.

Our Mission: By meeting people where they are and collaborating with others, PFLAG realizes its vision through:

- Support for families, allies and people who are LGBTQ
- Education for ourselves and others about the unique issues and challenges facing people who are LGBTQ
- Advocacy in our communities to change attitudes and create policies and laws that achieve full equality for people who are LGBTQ

My dear friend Maurie Davidson first informed me about PFLAG and invited me to attend my first meeting in May 2013, when I was conducting research for this book. The meeting was an amazing, eye-opening experience and it made me wish I had known about the group when I was younger and going through my own issues. I strongly encourage young people who are coming out to their families to go to these meetings and encourage their families to go as well. The parents were at the meeting to support their children, whether or not they understood as much as they would have liked. It is a process for everyone involved and I commend those parents for being very brave.

I particularly remember a woman from another country who attended and had found it difficult to accept her daughter's orientation because of her culture, but she was doing her best to be there for her daughter nonetheless. I also remember one of the mothers asking the group, "So many negative things kids hear about being gay, what are some of the positive things we can tell our children about being gay?" Although I had only planned on being there to observe, I surprised myself by answering her question. I said, "I think most people who are gay are more understanding or accepting of other people, of different cultures, religions etc., because they know what it's like to be different, to be made fun of. So in general, they have more compassion for others. They are more apt to understand and realize we are all really the same in spite of our differences."

It's funny how I had never really thought about it until I heard the question asked. Growing up, it seemed there were only negative things associated with being gay, and teens are already more prone to feeling bad about themselves even if they're straight. It's no wonder that the suicide rate is so high among gay teens. But as I've been highlighting throughout this book, the more organizations offering support, and the more TV programs, films, and books addressing the subject, the easier it's getting for everyone to accept and be accepted.

Family Equality Council

Family Equality Council is another strong organization offering tremendous support to the LGBTQ community. From their website:

"The Family Equality Council connects, supports, and represents the three million parents who are LGBT in this country, and their six million children. We are changing attitudes and policies to ensure that all families are respected, loved, and celebrated—including families with parents who are LGBT. We are a community of parents and children, grandparents and grandchildren that reaches across this country. For thirty years we have raised our children and raised our voices toward fairness for all families."

Why Family Equality Council is Needed

- Parents who are LGBT care about the same things all parents do—hugs and homework, bedtime, and bathtime.
- These moms and dads want the same things for their children that all parents do: respect, protection, celebration, and a bright future.
- These moms and dads are raising their children to love their country, stand up for their friends, treat others the way they would like to be treated, and tell the truth. The truth is society discriminates against these parents and their children, based on their parents' untraditional love for each other.
- Too often, the law treats these family members as strangers.
- Family Equality Council looks forward to a day when all families are valued for their commitment to each other.
- Moms and dads who are LGBT come together in a strong community that provides friendship,

good advice, and support—just like any other community of parents.

- Children with parents who are LGBT can meet, play, and make friends with other children who have LGBT moms and dads.
- LGBT men and women can find information on starting a family, adopting, or becoming foster parents—and children can find forever families.
- More Americans know a family with parents who are LGBT—and realize how much we all have in common.
- Children are safer from bullying.
- More schools, places of worship, hospitals and clinics, and government agencies treat families with parents who are LGBT with the respect that all families deserve.
- The law more often recognizes all the moms and dads who have made the commitment to be parents.
- We are creating a world where all loving families are recognized, respected, protected, and celebrated.

To find out more about Family Equality Council, go to http://www.familyequality.org.

GLAAD

The Gay & Lesbian Alliance Against Defamation is leading the conversation for LGBTQ equality and making big changes in the cultural landscape as the principal organization that works directly with news media, entertainment media, cultural institutions, and social media.

GLAAD's Mission: To amplify the voice of the LGBT community by empowering real people to share their stories, holding the media accountable for the words and images they present, and helping grassroots organizations communicate effectively. By ensuring that the stories of LGBT people are heard through the media, GLAAD promotes understanding, increases acceptance and advances equality.

GLSEN (pronounced *"lisen"*)
The Gay, Lesbian and Straight Education Network is an organization based in the United States and seeks to end discrimination, harassment, and bullying based on sexual orientation, gender identity, and gender expression in K–12 schools. GLSEN is headquartered in New York City and the District of Columbia. At the time of publication, there are currently forty chapters across the country representing cities, states, or regions. GLSEN supports gay-straight alliance, along with sponsoring the annual National Day of Silence and No Name-Calling Week, providing resources for teachers on how to support LGBT students, such as "Safe Schools" training. It also sponsors and participates in a host of other Days of Action, including TransAction Day, Ally Week, and the Martin Luther King, Jr. Organizing Weekend.

The following statement appears on GLSEN's official website:

There will be a new partnership to broaden inclusion of LGBT content in teacher preparation. GLSEN, the American Association of Colleges for Teacher Education

(AACTE) and the Association of Teacher Educators (ATE) are partnering on an effort to ensure that the next generation of teachers is equipped to effectively teach lesbian, gay, bisexual, and transgender (LGBT) youth, and to combat anti-LGBT bias in their schools. All too often, LGBT students and families face discrimination, stigmatization, and even violence in school. Supportive teachers can make a tremendous difference by creating safe classrooms and affirming curricula, but our research shows that many are not adequately prepared to address these issues in school.

Under this partnership, GLSEN, AACTE, and ATE will:

- Improve the knowledge base regarding the state of teacher preparation on LGBT issues through a national survey of teacher educators.
- Develop programmatic efforts and resources, informed by the research findings, to further inclusion of LGBT issues in teacher preparation.

Pop Luck Club

Based in West Hollywood, California, the Pop Luck Club is an all-volunteer, nonprofit organization launched and incorporated in 1998 by a group of gay men wanting to be parents. Today the group includes over 400 families raising more than 500 children. It is a close-knit community where many of the dads have been watching one another's kids grow up for years. Gay men who are considering becoming parents or who are beginning to take steps toward becoming dads continue to be welcomed and comprise a substantial portion of Pop Luck Club members. The organization helps arrange playdates, babysitters, recommendations for schools, and even offers guidance on issues such as how schoolteachers should handle Mother's Day in classrooms.

LifeWorks

LifeWorks is the youth development and mentoring program of the Los Angeles LGBT Center. The program offers one-on-one peer and group mentoring opportunities for lesbian, gay, bisexual, transgender, queer, and questioning youth, ages twelve to twenty-four. Their mission is to help LGBTQ youth realize their goals and dreams with the support of a safe space, positive and affirming role models, and workshops and activities that are fun and educational.

Chely Wright's LIKEME® Organization

The LIKEME Organization was founded in March 2010 by country music star Chely Wright after she made the conscious decision to publicly come out and advocate for the LGBTQ community. Wright also released her bestselling book, *Like Me*, a new album, and an award-winning documentary entitled *Wish Me Away* as she began her activism. She also currently serves as national spokesperson for GLSEN and appears regularly in the media to speak on LGBTQ equality and the needs of the LGBTQ community.

The LIKEME® organization states on their website that their mission is to provide a safe and welcoming space where LGBTQ individuals and their families, friends, and straight allies can come for education and resources, and to build a cohesive LGBTQ community in the Midwest. It speaks out at schools, colleges, corporations, and in the media about the need for LGBTQ equality, and speaks against classroom and LGBTQ bullying. They promote inclusion, respect, and equality for all the LGBTQ community and do so by meeting, knowing, supporting, and respecting all people.

The group prides itself in choosing to seek out the ways in which we might be similar rather than the ways we might be different, yet celebrates each other's individuality. LIKEME® is about being who you are meant to be. The organization has also taken it a step further with the Chely Wright LIKEME® Scholarship, which provides financial support for students pursuing a college degree and who actively advocate for LGBTQ youth and/or students severely affected by teen bullying or suicide of an LGBTQ youth. Through this scholarship, LGBTQ affected youth can apply for funding to pay for educational expenses to pursue a degree from an accredited college, university, or technical/vocational program. In 2014, LIKEME® awarded five scholarships for $1,250 each.

Out & Equal Workplace Advocates

Out & Equal is a United States nonprofit LGBTQ workplace equality organization, headquartered in San Francisco, California. The organization defines its vision as follows: "To achieve workplace equality for all regardless of sexual orientation, gender identity, expression, or characteristics." Out & Equal states its mission is to "Educate and empower organizations, human resource professionals, Employee Resource Groups (ERGs), and individual employees through programs and services that result in equal policies, opportunities, practices, and benefits in the workplace regardless of sexual orientation, gender

identity, expression, or characteristics." Out & Equal also provides training and sensitivity resources to LGBTQ employees
and corporations alike through advocacy, training programs,
and events.

Gay Dad Project

Founded by Amie Shea, the Gay Dad Project is not just limited to gay dads. It's a community with the purpose of enabling
everyone to communicate when a parent comes out. They are
putting together a documentary with the same name as the organization. Amie Shea is from Cut Bank, Montana, and attended
San Diego State University. I had the chance to interview her
by phone. She tells her story about growing up with a gay dad:

"During high school I knew my dad was gay, but I was completely terrified to talk about it with anyone then. At college
I was able to open up more about having a gay dad but I still
worried about the safety of my dad, our family, and what could
or would happen if anyone ever found out our family secret. My
hope is that the Gay Dad Project can help inspire and generate
meaningful conversations about sexuality and marriage in the
modern world. It is my sincere hope that the Gay Dad Project
will help expose the need for more acceptance and tolerance."

The documentary they are making will put names to faces,
and faces to the places of families who have experienced a parent coming out. It will introduce the audience to the gay parents, straight spouses, and children from various locations in
the United States, and possibly other parts of the world as well.
With people sharing their stories through interviews and on-
location footage, their hope is that the film will be a powerful
educational tool to let the world know that these families exist

and thrive. They hope it will also provide encouragement and support for people who may not be aware that there are other families like theirs. To learn more about the Gay Dad Project, go to http://www.gaydadproject.org/who-we-are/.

They are also putting together a book that will speak directly to children with gay parents and address certain issues such as: What it's like to find out one of your parents is gay? What emotions do you feel? How do you process it? How do your feelings change over time? Through a collaboration of writings from various children who were born to one gay parent and one straight parent, the book will also focus on the emotions and challenges of finding out one parent is gay, coping with the process, accepting the reality of the situation, and even embracing the uniqueness of having a gay parent. To find out more, go to http://gaydadproject.org/share-your-story/all-stories/.

Friends of Project 10

Friends of Project 10 was originally founded by Virginia Levy and Gayle Rolf with the vision to have LGBTQ students as fully included and affirmed in a public school environment where justice, equality, and respect for all prevail. With the mission to support programs which emphasize nondiscrimination and equality for LGBTQ youth, the organization also works to assure that public schools are in compliance with state and federal laws regarding sexual orientation and gender identity, and that academic achievement should not be limited by being part of a marginalized social group.

In 1994, Friends of Project 10 initially started its Models of Excellence scholarship program as a single award named in the memory of Peter Kaufman (the son of Alvin and Irene

Kaufman). As time passed, more commemorations were made and the name changed to Models of Excellence Scholarship competition. Now, the organization awards $1,000, $2,000, and $3,000 scholarships to senior high school students from southern California public, private, and parochial schools who have advanced the civil rights of the LGBTQ population, and plan to further their academic studies in higher education.*

To find out more about Friends of Project 10 and its various programs, go to www.friendsofproject10.org.

*Used with permission from the Friends of Project 10

CHAPTER 11

Recommended Reading and Viewing

Much of my research for this book came from conducting surveys and asking participants a variety of questions about their personal experiences. One important question I asked everyone was: *Do you know of any books or films that were helpful in regard to LGBTQ families and the topics we are discussing?* This chapter will cover many of the books, films, and television programs recommended by the people I interviewed throughout each chapter and a few of my own I came across. I also interviewed a few of the authors of the recommended reads as well. These books are helpful to all parents to start conversations and teach diversity while entertaining.

Books for Children

Heather Has Two Mommies and other children's books by Lesléa Newman

When I told my sister I was writing this book, she mentioned another book she had heard of called *Heather Has Two Mommies*.

When I googled the book's author, Lesléa Newman, I discovered she had grown up just a town over from where I grew up on Long Island. After reading her book, I was inspired to contact her to set up an interview and she was kind enough to oblige. Lesléa Newman is the author of more than fifty other books, including *A Letter to Harvey Milk*, *Nobody's Mother*, *Write from the Heart*, *The Boy Who Cried Fabulous*, *The Best Cat in the World*, *Still Life with Buddy*, and *Jail Bait*. She is a true pioneer who has been writing on this subject long before others dared to.

Heather Has Two Mommies was written in 1988 with the purpose of helping younger children (ages three to seven) with lesbian mothers. It was the first children's book to portray lesbian families in a positive way and to help them feel good about themselves and their families. Many schools still don't allow such books to be read in classrooms, as they feel such messages only devalue the traditional family unit. But Lesléa says it best in her book: "The most important thing about a family is that all the people in it love each other."

During our conversation, Lesléa discussed the feedback from her readers. She told me about a "lesbian Kodak moment," where after a lesbian mother had read *Heather Has Two Mommies* to her son, she immediately asked what he thought about it. The boy replied, "Can I get a dog or a cat?" Having two moms was obviously no big thing to this young boy. Then there are some of the other responses to the book she lists on her website:

- "There was the time Representative Robert Smith read portions of the book to the entire United States Senate, though no milk and cookies were served."

- "There was the time a man took the book off a public library shelf, went into the bathroom and defecated on it."
- "There were many instances when I was accused of writing a book that taught first graders the ins and outs of sodomy, no pun intended."
- "And there was that nasty 'no promo homo' bill which, if approved, would make reading *Heather Has Two Mommies* to a child without parental permission a felony. Luckily the bill never passed."

Two other books by Lesléa Newman and illustrated by Carol Thompson are *Mommy, Mama, and Me* and *Daddy, Papa, and Me*. These are the first board books ever published for kids who live in same-sex parent families. Both books depict a fun-filled day in the life of a happy, loving family.

One of her more current books is called *Donovan's Big Day* with illustrations by Mike Dutton. What I really like about this book is you can feel the excitement of little Donovan as he gets ready for something, but we don't know what yet. Lesléa captures the anticipation of little Donovan as he interacts with his family and does all the things he has to do to get ready for something big. We don't know until the end that it is to participate in the wedding of his two moms where he gets to be the ring bearer. It is a fun, beautifully written book, and shows, as many of her books do, that there are all kinds of families, and love is the most important thing. Look for her wonderful books at www.lesleakids.com.

Daddy's Roommate by Michael Willhoite

In recent years, there have been many other good books written specifically to be read to young children as a way to help break the ice and open up a discussion about having two moms or two dads. However, *Daddy's Roommate* was one of the first to portray gay life in a positive way and is another book that I highly recommend. What I especially like about it is that it portrays a gay couple to be not unlike everyone else and basically do the same things heterosexual couples do: take care of the house, argue, and spend time with their child.

Unfortunately, *Daddy's Roommate* was one of the most banned books by the American Library Association, which listed this book as number two on their list of the 100 most challenged books from 1990 to 2000 due to its subject matter and targeted audience.

Bob, The Lady Bug: Bob's New Pants

Tommy Starling is the author, illustrated by Jacquie Gonzalez. The story centers around Bob, a curious ladybug who learns he lives in a world of diversity and he is forced to learn and teach lessons of acceptance. The book was written for children ages three through seven, with the goal of helping children to accept diversity and ultimately end bullying. Del Shores was very impressed by the book, and said: "Tommy Starling has written a wonderful children's book that is so important and powerful. *Bob, The Ladybug: Bob's New Pants*, speaks to our times with a simple, beautiful message of acceptance and diversity, with Bob's determination to end bullying. Jacquie Gonzalez's illustrations are vibrant, beautiful, and captivating. Please share this amazing book with your children, your nieces and nephews, and all your friends! Well done, Tommy!"

It's Okay to Be Different and *The Family Book* by Todd Parr

These are excellent books for gay parents (or any parents) to read to young children. *It's Okay to Be Different* lets kids know it's okay to be silly and be themselves, and illustrates other things like how some people are in wheelchairs. It also lets kids know it's okay to have different families, like having two moms or two dads.

The Family Book lists different kinds of families, including single parents, stepparents, or same-sex parents. The section of the book dealing with same-sex parenting caused some controversy in the San Francisco Bay area, where the author did a reading at an elementary school. The students had to get permission slips to be read the book and two of them had to be escorted out when it got to the page about same-sex parents because their parents didn't want them hearing about that.

These two books are wonderful for children with two moms or two dads so that they feel more included and can feel their families are just as important as other families.

How It Feels to Have a Gay or Lesbian Parent (A Book by Kids for Kids of All Ages) by Judith E. Snow

This book expresses the feelings and experiences of children, teens, and young adults who have an LGBTQ parent. They speak openly about learning of their parent's sexual orientation and how it affected them and their families. They speak about prejudice and harassment, conflict and confusion, adaptation and adjustment, and hope for tolerance and a family that can exist in harmony. I like the fact that the kids were all ages, some only eight or ten, but they also spoke with adults who were in their twenties and thirties who were just finding out about their parents.

Children's Books That Tackle Trans

One interesting children's book about transgender people that I came across is called *Backwards Day* by S. Bear Bergman. It tells a story about the planet Tenalp, where one day each year, boys turn into girls and girls turn into boys. One year a girl named Andrea doesn't change back to a She the day after Backwards Day, and his parents take him to consult with the "Backwardologists" who help them to understand what is happening.

Another good children's book that deals with this subject is *The Adventures of Tulip, Birthday Wish Fairy*, also by S. Bear Bergman. It's about Tulip, a birthday wish fairy who grants wishes to all the nine-year-olds in North America. When Tulip comes across David, a boy who wishes to live as Daniela, it's a request he's never had before, so he asks the Wish Fairy Captain for advice.

Both of the above stories are told with understanding and compassion, but what I also really appreciated was their humor, which you don't see a lot in books about LGBTQ families.

BOOKS FOR LGBTQ PARENTS

Does This Baby Make Me Look Straight? by Dan Bucatinsky

As you can probably guess by the title, this book is written with a great sense of humor and addresses the concerns some people have with questions like "How important is it for a child to

have a mom?"; "What is the child missing by not having one?"
Even as a gay man, I have to admit I've had my own concerns
about a child having same-sex parents. Although I know the
most important thing is for a child to be loved and brought up
with solid values, the questions have always gnawed at me. But
as I read through this book, my concerns gradually eased as
when I also did my own research and spoke with people from
the different families portrayed.

Stuck in The Middle with You: A Memoir of Parenting in Three Genders by Jennifer Finney Boylan

I highly recommend this book for families with a transgender parent. It is a true story about the author coming out as transgender
when her two children were young. As she transitioned from a
man to a woman and from a father to a mother, Jennifer's family
dealt with unique and hard challenges and answered many tough
questions for themselves. This memoir also does an excellent job of
showing what makes one family more complicated than another.

Loving Someone Gay by Don Clark

One of the therapists I interviewed told me about this book,
originally published in 1977. I read the revised version (published in 1987) and although it was still a little dated, I found it
to be very helpful in determining the real pros and cons for kids
with gay parents.

Is It a Choice? by Eric Marcus

This is actually one of the first books I read about being gay and
I highly recommend it for any relative just being introduced to

the idea of a having a gay family member. The book answers 300 of the most frequently asked questions about gays and lesbians. It addresses issues such as religion, how kids react to having gay parents, what gay bars are like, why people are fighting for the legal right to get married, and many more important topics. Although the latest edition of his book was written in 2005 and much has changed since that time, the core of it offers excellent advice that will always remain the same. Eric has also written a version of *Is It a Choice?* specifically for teens and their parents called *What If?* For more information, visit www.ericmarcus.com.

Families Like Mine by Abigail Garner

Highly recommended. The book had many helpful stories. In the book, Abby shares her own story of finding out her father was gay. She was glad it was when she was younger: "I could have easily adopted some of the homophobic attitudes that are prevalent in our society. If that had happened, I would have had to come to terms with my dad being gay rather than simply accepting it."

A few other books recommended by those I interviewed were:

- *Sometimes the Spoon Runs Away with Another Spoon,* children's coloring book by Jacinta Bunnell, recommended by Dr. Kotulski
- *My Uncle's Wedding,* by Eric Ross, recommended by Dr. Kotulski
- *Confessions of a Fairy's Daughter: Growing Up with a Gay Dad* by Alison Wearing, recommended by Amie Shea

- *This Is How You Say Goodbye: A Daughter's Memoir* by
  Victoria Loustalot, recommended by Amie Shea.
  This is How You Say Goodbye is about a father taking
  his daughter on a trip around the globe, though
  the daughter is unaware that her father is dying of
  AIDS.
- Three books published by PFLAG: *The ABC's
  of Gender*, *Dragonfly Stories*, and a book on
  crossdressing called *My Husband Wears My Clothes*.

Recommended Movies and TV

Some of these films, TV shows, and documentaries are for
adults just to get a better understanding of different subjects
and some are good for the whole family to watch.

Hollywood To Dollywood

I recommend this documentary to families to help break the ice
when coming out to other family members and, of course, to
Dolly Parton fans. The film came out a few years ago and it follows identical twins Gary and Larry Lane as they embark on an
adventure and drive their rented RV (named Jolene) across the
country from Hollywood to Tennessee, and then to Dollywood
to hand Dolly Parton a script they had written for her. The film
won over twenty-five documentary awards and features fifteen
Dolly Parton songs (that alone is worth owning the movie).

The documentary also shows the twins revealing that they
are gay, which was unknown to many of their family and friends
in their conservative hometown in North Carolina. The twins
meet many interesting characters along the way, including their

friends Leslie Jordan, Chad Allen, and Ann Walker. I absolutely love this film and I was even more moved by it the second time I watched it. I had the opportunity to interview Gary and Larry, who a few years previously had won the top prizes in two popular TV reality shows, *Fear Factor* and *Wipeout*. However, I mostly spoke to them about the impact of the film and asked for their advice on speaking to children about LGBTQ relatives. They told me about a nineteen-year-old from Minnesota who had contacted them after seeing the movie and revealed his plan to post on Facebook that he was about to watch the movie with his parents and then come out to them afterward.

Another interesting moment was at a film festival during the Q&A following the screening of the documentary. A woman in the audience shared that her fifteen-year-old son had come out to her the day before and, with today being his birthday, he wanted to see the movie with her. The twins have also been contacted by the principal at their former high school, as well as several of the teachers and hometown residents who have all expressed their support and pride in this courageous film. However, the issue is still not really discussed in their own family, and being Southern Baptist, it is extremely hard to break through their religious mind-set.

The lack of conversation on this topic is something that is quite common. Not talking about it is how many families deal with it, but I believe this film will help some families to start the conversation. I also asked Larry and Gary at what age they thought this subject should be addressed with children. They both agreed between thirteen and fifteen years old, when the birds and bees are usually discussed, because before that kids probably won't fully understand and therefore it doesn't matter anyway. Kids love their uncles and aunts, and their uncles and aunts love them. Gary and Larry also used their celebrity to become major advocates for the "No Hate" campaign against Prop 8. Their film continues to help many people who see it.

Prayers for Bobby

Gary and Larry told me that they both found this movie to be very helpful and so, trusting their advice, I found a copy and watched it. It is a 2009 Lifetime movie, based on a true story, and stars Sigourney Weaver as Mary Griffith, who became a gay rights crusader after her teenage son committed suicide because of her religious intolerance. The film is based on the book of the same title by Leroy Aarons. Sigourney Weaver's performance was amazing, as was the entire cast. I found it to be one of the most moving films I have seen.

The Kids Are All Right

This 2010 award-winning film is one of the first to show a same-sex parent family. It is kind of a dark comedy, written and directed by Lisa Cholodenko. Nic (Annette Bening) and Jules (Julianne Moore) shine in the roles as the parents of two teenage children. All heck breaks loose when the biological father of their children, played brilliantly by Mark Ruffalo, comes into their lives after their son finds the sperm donor for him and his sister. I thought this film did an excellent job of portraying the situation in such a realistic human way. It showed that no families, no parents, and no person is perfect, not even those who pretend to be.

Documentaries

That's a Family!

That's a Family! is another excellent documentary from the late Debra Chasnoff, who also made *It's Elementary: Talking About Gay Issues in School.* In the film, children from diverse families, including many with different races and religions, and some with LGBTQ parents, talk about what they would like other kids to know about their family structures. It's only thirty-five minutes long, but full of powerful messages that help to prevent prejudice and embrace diversity. It also does an excellent job of communicating to a young audience in a very entertaining way. I strongly recommend it as a must-see for every child and you can easily access it from New Day Film's website: https://www .newday.com/film/thats-family.

One of the questions asked in *That's a Family!* was "What makes a good family?" Some of my favorite responses were:
- "Everyone needs to take care of each other, feel comfortable with each other, and feel trust and friendliness."
- "If you have just one parent and you get in trouble, only one person gets mad and only one person nags at you, so I think I am pretty lucky."
- "The only bad thing about having two moms is that sometimes kids use mean words for gays and lesbians and that hurts my feelings. I wish they knew it is okay to have two moms or two dads. It's okay to be different."

In My Shoes

COLAGE put out this excellent short film called *In My Shoes*, a thirty-minute documentary by and about children of lesbian, gay, bisexual, and transgender parents with an informative portrayal of many types of LGBTQ families. The film won the Audience Award for Best Short at the San Francisco International LGBTQ Film Festival in 2005. Directed, shot, and edited by Jen Gilomen, it has an ending that has a powerful message: "It doesn't matter if you agree with my family. What matters is if you give us respect and equal rights."

Becoming Chaz

Becoming Chaz is an interesting documentary about being transgender. It features Chaz Bono, the transgender child of Sonny and Cher, and his transition. Not only was the film popular because of the celebrity factor, but it was also very well done. In the film, Chaz says, "Young people seem to get it; the youngest person in my family got this immediately." Chaz explained that older people, like his mom, Cher, took quite a bit of time to adjust. Cher said that what helped her understand a little more was for her to think about if she woke up one day in a man's body and how she would feel the need to get out of it as quickly as possible because she loves being a woman.

Two Spirits

Released in 2009, this documentary tells the story of a transgender Navajo teen killed in a brutal hate crime in 2001. One of the film's subjects talks about the Navajo culture and says, "It basically teaches to accept people for who they are, how they present to us, and we only judge them on the basis of what did they contribute to the human society, how do they treat their children, how do they treat their elders." I found his statement to be brilliant in its simplicity and I personally believe this rule should be adopted by all cultures, all religions, and all people.

Southern Comfort

A 2001 documentary about a trans man who developed ovarian cancer and was refused medical treatment because he was transgender. The film documents the final year of his life.

Documentaries on Religion

Fish Out of Water

Pastor Jerrell Walls recommended the 2009 documentary *Fish out of Water* because it specifically focuses on the subject of Bible verses and homosexuality. Written and directed by Ky Dickens, the film addresses the seven Bible verses that condemn homosexuality and justify discrimination against same-sex marriage. If you're like me, you will also really appreciate how the filmmaker uses humor and original animation to make a traditionally complex and controversial topic accessible to those who don't like talking about religion and sexuality. The film also speaks to hundreds of gay, lesbian, bisexual, and transgender folks and asks them to talk about their experiences with their faith and sexuality.

For the Bible Tells Me So

Another great documentary Jerrell Walls and Chely Wright recommended is *For the Bible Tells Me So* (2009), directed by Daniel G. Karslake and cowritten with Helen R. Mendoza. It talks about religion and homosexuality in the US and how the religious right has used its interpretation of the Bible to demonize gay people. One of the more touching stories in the film is about a mother who could not accept her daughter's orientation until it was too late. Because of her religious beliefs, she rejected her gay daughter. Only after her daughter committed suicide did she begin to read books on the subject and talk to other people, eventually becoming a crusader for gay rights. So sad that it took her daughter's death to wake her up.

Television Shows

Degrassi: The Next Generation

On the cable channel Teen Nick Television, there is a series called *Degrassi: The Next Generation*, which was attacked by the Florida Family Association (FFA). The show first aired in 2001 and portrayed controversial issues like school shootings, teen pregnancy, homosexuality, cutting, and STD outbreaks, among others. In one of the episodes, a student in junior high school finds out her father is gay. It was done very realistically. The show really covered a lot in a half-hour episode. The shock when she found out, then anger toward her dad for not telling her earlier and also for being selfish and leaving the family for another man. When a friend of hers suggested her father might be gay she became really offended, thought she was making a bad joke, threw a drink at her, and stormed off. It turned out the friend's brother was gay and she was just trying to help.

There was a lot of controversy about another episode titled "My Body Is A Cage," a two-part episode about a transgender student that won a Peabody Award. I watched it and found it very realistic and well done, especially the way some of the boy bullies shove the female-to-male transgender student out of the bathroom. One of his girlfriends, upon finding out, says "I've seen you freaks on Oprah." The mother has a hard time accepting it, saying, "You made such a pretty girl." Then the child said, "But I was never happy." His mom replied, "I just don't understand," and the child says, "You don't have to. Just accept."

Shows like these open up the dialogue among kids and allow them to feel more comfortable in being themselves. Perhaps it enables them to be more accepted by fellow students instead of being bullied. Liz Owen, director of communications for PFLAG, said that both the TV series and PFLAG's intention was to educate teens about transgender classmates in order to prevent bullying. "The episode acknowledges that there are trans people out there and due to bullying and harassment in a school setting, they really have a hard time," Owen said. "Our message boards got overwhelmingly positive feedback from trans kids saying how much it helped them, and from other kids saying that while they didn't have any transgender kids in their school, they would act positively if they did."

Buddy G, My Two Moms and Me
In my research, I came across a cartoon from 2007 called *Buddy G, My Two Moms and Me*, created by Margaux Towne. What a great way to teach kids about diversity—through a cartoon!

Buddy G was one of the first children's animated cartoon series starring a character with two parents of the same gender. It was entertaining and educational. The website to order the DVD is www.buddyg.com. You can also find them on Facebook.

Cartoons have come a long way since I watched Bugs Bunny as a kid, though Bugs did dabble a bit in cross-dressing as I recall, and I think he French-kissed Elmer Fudd once. Oh, that wascally wabbit!

Orange Is the New Black

The recent Netflix series about female prison inmates has become extremely popular for a number of reasons, but it's also one of the first programs to feature a transgender actress. This show is definitely not for kids to watch—or very conservative adults, for that matter. Laverne Cox plays an inmate who was born male and transitions to female. In one episode she has a flashback, revealing that although her wife had been very supportive, her son, who was about eight years old at the time, did not take it very well. He was embarrassed but trying to accept it. The flashback shows them shopping for sneakers for the son when they run into a former coworker and friend of the father. Realizing that he is now a woman, the friend uncomfortably rushes off and this makes the son feel even worse about his dad. This episode did an excellent job of portraying some of the things transgender people go through and was a good way to help people gain a better understanding. Later on in season two, the son does come to visit his dad in prison and they finally break the ice by playing a card game together.

Transparent

The show *Transparent* is a very modern half-hour comedy on Amazon Prime which premiered in 2014 and features a family man played by Jeffrey Tambor who finally accepts being transgender and transitions into a woman. The show has won many awards, including Golden Globes, SAGs, and Emmys. Fair warning: it's not a show for the whole family to watch. It's a little racy for kids under a certain age, even for some adults, I'd imagine. But it definitely shows some of the struggles for those transitioning, especially at a later age.

While these books, films, and TV programs all deal with LGBTQ issues, there are also two films that were highly recommended to me for teaching people about acceptance in general. *La Vie en Rose* (2007) is a great film about acceptance and embracing all with love, and *Billy Elliot* (2000) is for anyone of any age to learn about accepting anyone for who they are. I am sure the next few years will have even more inspiring, entertaining, and educational films and books by, for, and about the LGBTQ community.

CHAPTER 12

We've Come a Long Way:
The Last Mile Is Always the Longest

"Acceptance has got to start in the home."

That is from Michael Bublé's interview with Thomas Howard Jr. on November 12, 2010, on MatthewsPlace.com, a site designed to help young people gain the skills and tools to lead healthy, productive, hate-free lives. Bublé also said, "My uncle Mike has been with my uncle Frank, they've been a couple for thirty-five years. So when I grew up, my mom and dad, in no uncertain terms, said, you know, 'Michael, a man can be in love with a man and a woman can be in love with a woman, and there's no difference between people that are gay or straight. They're born that way. It's not something that can be learned or unlearned, or it's not a phase or anything like that. This is something that you are born with.' And so I grew up never seeing a difference between gay and straight people."

It can take a long time to write a book. I worked on this for quite a few years, and I was partly hoping there would no longer be a need for this book by the time I finally finished it. Time is changing attitudes that quickly. I noticed at a Gay Pride parade a few years ago that there were only a few people protesting with antigay signs. Fifteen or twenty years ago, there were certainly enough to "rain on the parade." However, there are still those people who carry the meanest, most spiteful signs of all, like "Jesus Hates Gays" or "God Doesn't Love You the Way You Are." Chely Wright's minister and spiritual advisor, Rev. Dr. C. Welter Gaddy, says in the documentary *Wish Me Away*, "There's no one as mean as someone who's mean for Jesus."

LGBTQ Legalities: Your Family Is Now Equal

A prequel to the historic Supreme Court ruling on same-sex marriage in 2015 was in June 2013, when the California Supreme Court ruled Prop 8 unconstitutional and unlocked the door for the legalization of same-sex marriage. Chris Perry and Sandy Sear were the plaintiffs in that suit and I was very moved when I saw them in a news conference on TV saying how happy they were that now all children are equal no matter what family you are in. In 2015, the Supreme Court made same-sex marriage legal in all fifty states.

Not so Fast

Following the 2015 ruling, some states enacted constitutional or statutory bans on same-sex marriage, known as "Defense of Marriage" Acts. But at least it is legal in all the states. You know what else had been legal in many states? Firing someone for being gay! At the time of publication, an employee can still be fired just for being gay in twenty-eight states, and in thirty states employees could have been fired for being transgender. So in essence, the children who live in these states and have parents or relatives that are LGBTQ were severely affected by such laws, as were families' entire financial situations, among other things. However, the LGBTQ community did have a victory in March 2017 when the US Seventh Circuit Court Of Appeals ruled 8–3 that you can't be fired for being gay. They found that workplace discrimination based on sexual orientation violates Title VII of the 1964 Civil Rights Act.

Don't Ask, Don't Tell Repealed

Until 2011, the "Don't Ask, Don't Tell" policy said that gay people couldn't openly serve in the military. Now they can, which is great, but when I spoke with John Dennem, he told me his nineteen-year-old nephew was serving in the army. Despite the fact that "Don't Ask, Don't Tell" had been repealed and gays and lesbians are supposed to be able to openly serve in the military, his nephew hears many negative and derogatory comments about gay people from his superiors. The young man also feels that he can't really say anything without putting his career or his own well-being at risk. His uncle, whom he loves very much, is gay, and yet he feels he has to put up with this. What kind of message does that send to young people? Someone is willing to lay down his or her life for a country of strangers but they're not supposed to love their own family member? How much more confusing can this be for a young person?

Antigay Discriminatory Laws

Recent legislation shows that we still have a long way to go.

In 2014, the Arizona Legislature passed a measure that allowed business owners asserting their religious beliefs to refuse service to gays and others. The 33–27 vote by the House sent the legislation to Governor Jan Brewer, a Republican. Similar religious protection legislation was introduced that year in Ohio, Kansas, Mississippi, Idaho, South Dakota, Tennessee, and Oklahoma, but Arizona's plan was the only one that passed. Some Republicans claim it is a First Amendment issue. Democrats say it is an outright attack on the rights of gays and lesbians. Many, the author of this book included, believe that these kinds of bills will encourage discrimination against the LGBTQ community.

Kansas, We Aren't in the 1800s Anymore

On February 23, 2014, the Kansas House of Representatives actually passed a bill allowing refusal of service to same-sex couples. It was officially called House Bill 2453 and it explicitly protects religious individuals, groups, and businesses that refuse services to same-sex couples, and particularly to those looking to tie the knot. The bill was not supported by the Kansas Senate.

Indiana

In March 2015, Governor Mike Pence of Indiana (vice president as of 2017) signed into law the state's Religious Freedom Restoration Act. The action drew sharp criticism and a major national backlash from people across the United States. The new law would allow businesses in the state of Indiana to cite religious objections and refuse service to gay people. While it's saddening to know that such a law would still be able to pass in this day and age, the overwhelming objection by American citizens does show that the majority of people's attitudes are changing.

Another good sign of change is the intense criticism from major corporations like Apple, Walmart, and tech giant Salesforce, who rallied against Indiana's law and similar measures advancing in at least a dozen other states. For instance, the NCAA, which was set to host its men's basketball Final Four in Indianapolis, said it would move their future events elsewhere. Even governors from other states called for boycotts in Indiana. Within three days of the bill's signing, at least $40 million of the state's economic activity was lost.

More LGBTQ People in Film and TV

Today, thanks in part to TV shows now portraying a lot more LGBTQ characters, being gay is not as big a deal as it used to be.

A good example is the TV show *Modern Family*, which includes a gay couple raising a child. It is a top-rated show that has been popular for many seasons now. Even Mitt Romney's wife, Ann, said it was one of her favorite shows when her husband was running for president on a very conservative platform.

TV shows such as *Modern Family* and another recent show, *The New Normal*, which was about a gay couple who want a baby, make the subject much easier for real life families today. The success of *Will & Grace* as a well-written comedy set the stage for other LGBTQ-themed programs to be welcomed into mainstream popular culture. I am very happy the show was brought back to life in 2017 for additional episodes. *Glee* is another award-winning series that has brought much awareness to the younger demographics as well. Other shows such as *Scandal* and *How to Get Away with Murder* also feature LGBTQ characters. On cable shows, LGBTQ people are featured even more—Showtime's *Shameless* (if you ever feel your family is screwed up, watching this show may ease some of those fears) has some gay characters and they did a few episodes with transgender characters as well. This show is not for kids to watch either. Netflix's *Sense 8* also featured gay, transgender characters (not for kids either).

We didn't have anything close to these kinds of shows growing up; instead, we watched families such as on *The Brady Bunch*, which never involved any gay characters or dealt with the topic at all. In fact, Robert Reed, who played Mike Brady (the father), was secretly gay. It was something he had to hide in his personal life throughout his many years on the show.

I later learned that Dick Sargent, the second actor to play Darrin Stephens on *Bewitched*, was "twinkling his toes" while Sam was "twinkling her nose." (Don't mind my politically incorrect humor; it's a result of watching way too much *Family Guy*.) I should also add that Paul Lynde, who played Samantha's Uncle Arthur, was gay, and Hayden Rorke, the actor on *I Dream of Jeannie* who played Dr. Bellows, also liked fellows. I believe it would have been much easier for me growing up gay had I known there were so many gay actors on the very shows I watched and enjoyed so much.

As I've shown in various examples throughout this book, there are more LGBTQ characters portrayed in film and TV than ever before. The Oscar for best movie of the year in 2017 went to *Moonlight*, which had a prominent gay theme to it.

One great example of how things are changing in media is a show on the Freeform network, which is geared to a younger demographic. One of their biggest shows right now is *The Fosters*, a show about a lesbian couple raising their five children, both biological and adopted. It's been on for several seasons. I love this show. The acting is great and the storylines are very realistic. Hopefully the show educates people who don't know families like these, and makes them realize that they are just like any other families, faults and all.

We've Come a Long Way

The 56th annual televised Grammy Awards show in 2014 showed an amazing, powerful performance of Macklemore's song "Same Love," where thirty-three gay and straight couples took the stage and said "I do" in a marriage ceremony performed by Queen Latifah. Perhaps even more important was the overwhelming positive response from viewers following the broadcast. However, we've still got . . .

A Long Way to Go

The historic mass wedding on the Grammys wasn't enjoyed by all. There were several antigay protestors who flocked to Twitter to spew their hateful views. Many claimed that the performance was nothing but a mockery of traditional marriage, Christianity, and family values. I read some of the homophobic tweets following the "Same Love" performance and many said how "sick" or "disgusting" it was, or how it was supposed to be a family-friendly show. One tweet said, "Maybe next year they can perform mass abortions," and another said, "Quit shoving your leftist agenda down our throats."

Even Disney Shows are Becoming More Progressive

The 2017 family-friendly Disney show *Good Luck Charlie* featured an episode with two lesbian moms. Interestingly, this groundbreaking episode aired on the same night as the 56th Grammy Awards in 2014. In the storyline, parents Amy and Bob Duncan (Leigh-Allyn Baker and Eric Allan Kramer) set up a playdate for their preschooler, Charlie (Mia Talerico), with one of her new pals, who happened to have two mothers. Not surprisingly, the conservative group One Million Moms (the same group that called for a boycott of JC Penney after the company partnered with Ellen DeGeneres) complained about the episode in a letter and said that the topic was too complicated for children to understand. Really? The show made it very simple to understand, so simple that a child could understand, in fact. Showing these kinds of modern families on these shows will help people become more familiar with them, understand them, and be more comfortable.

Transgender Homecoming Queen

Recently, I heard about a transgender teen named Cassidy Lynn Campbell, who was crowned homecoming queen at a California high school. She was so happy that the school recognized her for the gender she is.

Campbell is not the first transgender girl to be named homecoming queen of an educational institution in the United States. In 2009, Jesse Vasold received the title at William & Mary in Williamsburg, Virginia. Regardless of who came first, we've certainly come a long way if high school students are not only accepting their transgender fellow classmates but also giving them the ultimate honor of crowning them homecoming queen.

We may have come a long way, but there were some negative reactions to Campbell's win, so we have a ways to go. I think in time there will be fewer people who feel the need to say negative things about LGBTQ people.

Transgender Bathroom Law Controversy

In 2016, North Carolina passed a law to restrict public restroom use to the gender listed on a person's birth certificate. This got a lot of people's bowels in an uproar, as Archie Bunker used to say. There was a lot of backlash over this law that cost the state a lot of business—Bruce Springsteen even canceled a concert there. Several other states passed similar laws leading to a lot of controversy. These laws were passed based on irrational fears that transgender people are predators or will molest children. This is not true. These laws are just another form of discrimination. These laws show that we have a long way to go in letting people *go* where they feel most comfortable.

However, we've come a long way in that more people and more companies are coming to the defense of the LGBTQ community.

The Target chain made headlines when they said they would allow transgender customers to use the bathroom and fitting room that best aligns with that person's gender identity. This prompted boycotts, angry tweets, and some funny Facebook memes. But again, free publicity and promotion for Target from them.

Trump's Transgender Tweet

In July 2017, President Donald Trump tweeted that the US military would not accept transgender people, saying their service would cause "tremendous medical costs and disruption. After consultation with my Generals and military experts, please be advised that the United States Government will not accept or allow transgender individuals to serve in any capacity in the U.S. Military." This caused a lot of controversy as there were already thousands of transgender service members in the military. Subsequent court decisions have determined that transgender people may continue to serve.

Historic LGBTQ Election Wins of 2017

- Andrea Jenkins, an openly trans woman, was elected to the city council of Minneapolis.
- Danica Roem was elected to Virginia House of Delegates, becoming Virginia's first openly trans candidate to serve in a state legislature.
- Jenny Durkan was elected Mayor of Seattle, becoming the first openly lesbian mayor.

Freedom of Speech but Not at High School Graduation

In 2015, school officials in Colorado banned a high school valedictorian's commencement speech in which he planned to come out as gay. Eighteen-year-old Evan Young had wanted to publicly declare his sexual orientation during his graduation from the Twin Peaks Charter Academy in Longmont. Young went public to say school officials had barred him from speaking and did not acknowledge him as the senior class valedictorian.

The story had a little bit of a happy ending when Young got to give part of the speech when he appeared on *The Nightly Show with Larry Wilmore* in June 2015. His speech was put online and it went viral. An excerpt from the speech: "Since we're never going to see each other again, I thought I should share some of my deepest, darkest secrets . . . my biggest secret of all [is] I'm gay," said Young. "I understand this might be offensive to some people, but it's who I am."

How school officials in Colorado thought this was offensive and banned it is beyond me. Yes, we have a long way to go.

We've Come a Long Way . . . Toward a Touchdown

In 2013, a defensive lineman from the University of Missouri, Michael Sam, spoke publicly about his sexual orientation. In 2014, he became the first openly gay player drafted to the National Football League and was chosen by the St. Louis Rams. The controversy erupted and all hell broke loose when he kissed his boyfriend on national TV. Some people took to Twitter, furiously tweeting their disgust . . . long way to go.

2014 Russian Olympics

In June 2013, Russian president Vladimir Putin signed into law a bill banning the "propaganda of nontraditional sexual relations to minors," which limits the rights of the country's lesbian, gay, bisexual, transgender, and intersex people. Article 6.21 says: "Propaganda is the act of distributing information among minors that (1) is aimed at the creating nontraditional sexual attitudes, (2) makes nontraditional sexual relations attractive, (3) equates the social value of traditional and nontraditional sexual relations, or (4) creates an interest in nontraditional sexual relations."

Putin declared in a TV interview that the law was aimed at banning propaganda of homosexuality and pedophilia, suggesting that gays are more likely to abuse children. The law on propaganda has also been used to justify barring gay pride rallies on the grounds that children might see them. Many wondered how athletes and fans would be treated for any gay rights protestation during the Olympics. Putin then accused the United States of having double standards in its criticism of Russia, referencing laws that remain on the books in some US states classifying gay sex as a crime. The US Supreme Court, however, ruled in 2003 that such laws were unconstitutional. Homosexuality was a crime in the entire former Soviet Union, which collapsed in 1991. It was decriminalized in Russia in 1993. However, in 2017 concentration camps for homosexuals were opened in Chechnya, where electric shock torture was used on gay men and many were beaten to death. So two steps forward . . . a thousand steps back.

Uganda Be Kidding

Even with some setbacks and some hurdles to still clear here in the United States for LGBTQ people, things are still better here than in other parts of the world. In 2017, there was a bill signed in Uganda that further bans homosexuality. The bill was originally named "Kill the Gays" and went as far as calling for the death penalty for certain homosexual acts. They changed it after an international uproar. Currently the bill states anyone who conducts marriage ceremonies for same-sex couples faces seven years behind bars. Failure to report homosexual activity to police is also criminalized. Doctors who treat gays, landlords who rent them property, and those suspected of being LGBTQ are subject to five-year prison terms under the bill. Anyone who offers support to homosexuals will also be committing a criminal offense. Needless to say, I won't be vacationing in Uganda anytime soon.

President Obama Signs Executive Order

June 2014 marked a huge victory for equality. The White House announced it would protect 16 million more Americans from discrimination in the workplace. President Barack Obama signed an executive order that provides protections to people working for federal contractors nationwide who could face job discrimination because of their gender identity or sexual orientation.

Moving Forward/Moving Backward

Changes are occurring faster than I can write. Some good, some bad. Some moving forward, some moving backward. In November 2017, Australia voted yes to same-sex marriage by more than 61 percent in a two-month national postal survey. Moving forward. Transgender candidates were elected for the first time in 2017 in places like central India and Montreal. Moving forward. But also around that same time, Ankara, the capital of Turkey, banned public showings of LGBTQ films and exhibitions. Moving backward. I find this disturbing partly because I am part Turkish.

In Closing

I hope the stories and advice in this book have been helpful. While much of the advice from my interviewees fell along the same lines, some was also contradictory, which goes to show that every single family and relationship is different; everyone has to decide what is best for them. For example, the majority of people I spoke with felt that younger is better to start having the conversations with kids. I believe that is good advice to keep in mind, even though a few parents suggested waiting until they are a little older. Some say it's better to tell all the kids at the same time so none are harboring a secret, while some say to wait.

Many of the stories emphasize teaching children to treat everyone equally and showing that love is the most important thing in a family. These simple things should offset any negative words the child is hearing on media or elsewhere.

In this book, we may have been a little general in some areas and some issues we just touched upon briefly. For those who may have more serious issues that may need addressing, please continue your research with additional books or articles that deal with specific subjects of concern in more depth or seek the advice of a professional.

I found a lot of irony in the writing of this book because it seemed as though some adults were more likely to have issues than the kids. Through my research and interviews, I can see great strides are being made for LGBTQ people, and though some problems do still exist, more and more past issues are now nonissues.

When I was a kid, our family used to drive from Long Island to the Adirondack Mountains to visit relatives. It took about six hours. My mother would always say, "The last mile is the longest." I really hope we don't have too many more miles to go before being LGBTQ is not an issue at all and everyone is treated fairly based upon their actions rather than their sexual status. The ultimate destination is where we can all just live together with our differences and everyone can just be who they are. The time when we finally do not hate people because we do not understand them or simply because they are different. Writing this book has been a journey for me, and I truly hope it will help us to take another step in the right direction.

Resources

Books:

Berman S, Bear and K.D. Diamond. *Backwards Day*. Toronto: Flamingo Rampant, 2012.

Berman, S. Bear and Suzy Malik. *The Adventures Of Tulip, Birthday Wish Fairy*. Toronto: Flamingo Rampant, 2012.

Boyle, Jennifer. *Stuck In The Middle With You (A Memoir Of A Parent In Two Genders)*. New York: Crown, 2013.

Bucatinsky, Dan. *Does This Baby Make Me Look Straight? Confessions Of A Gay Dad*. New York: Touchstone, 2012.

Clarke, Don. *Loving Someone Gay*. New Jersey: Lethe Press, 1976.

Corley, Rip. *The Final Closet: The Gay Parents Guide For Coming Out To Children*. Miami: Editech Press, 1990.

Fairchild, Betty and Nancy Hayward. *Now That You Know About Homosexuality, A Parents' Guide To Understanding Their Gay And Lesbian Children*. Florida: Harcourt, Brace & Company, 1979.

Garner, Abigail. *Families Like Mine*. New York: HarperCollins, 2004.

Marcus, Eric. *Is It A Choice?* New York: HarperCollins, 1993.

Miller, Stuart Howell. *Prayer Warriors, the true story of a gay son, his fundamentalist Christian family and the Battle For His Soul.* New York: Alyson Books, 1999.

Newman, Lesléa. *Donovan's Big Day.* New York: Tricycle Press, 2011.

Newman, Lesléa. *Heather Has Two Mommies.* New York: Alyson Books, 2000.

Parr, Todd. *It's Okay to Be Different.* Boston: Little, Brown & Co., 2001.

Parr, Todd. *The Family Book.* New York: Little Brown Books For Young Readers, 2003.

Parnell, Peter, Justin Richardson and Henry Cole. *And Tango Makes Three.* New York: Simon & Shuster Children's Publishing, 2005.

Ross, Eric. *My Uncle's Wedding.* Createspace Independent Publishing Platform, 2011.

Snow, Judith. E. *How It Feels To Have a Gay or Lesbian Parent, A Book by Kids for Kids of all Ages.* London: Routeledge, Taylor and Francis Group, 2004.

Starling, Tommy and Jackie Gonzalez. *Bob The LadyBug, Bob's New Pants.* Bob The LadyBug Publishing, 2012.

Willhoite, Michael. *Daddy's Roomate.* New York: Alyson Books,1991.

Wright, Chely. *Like Me, Confessions of a Heartland Country Singer.* New York: Pantheon, 2010.

MOVIES/TV:

Becoming Chaz, directed by Fenton Bentley and Randy Barbato, World Of Wonder Productions (2011).

Buddy G My Two Moms & Me, created by Margaux Towne, Us2 Productions (2007).

Bully, directed by Lee Hirsch, Bully Project (2011).

Degrassi: The Next Generation, various directors, Bell Broadcast & New Media Fund (2001-2015).

The Nightly Show, Evan Young's Banned Graduation Speech, Comedy Central (2015) https://www.youtube.com/watch?v=0T-kazH0XPk

Fish Out Of Water, directed by Ky Dickens, Yellow Wing Productions (2009).

For The Bible Tells Me So, directed by Daniel Karslake, Atticus Group (2007).

The Fosters, created by Peter Paige and Bradley Bredweg, Blazing Elm Entertainment (2013).

Good Luck Charlie, created by Phil Baker and Drew Vaupen, It's A Laugh Productions (2013).

Hollywood To Dollywood, directed by John Lavin, Bloodrush Films (2011).

In My Shoes, directed by Jen Gilomen, COLAGE (2005).

I Now Pronounce You Chuck and Larry, directed by Dennis Dugan, Universal Pictures (2007).

It's Elementary, directed by Debra Chasnoff and Helen Cohen, Groundspark (1996).

The Kids Are All Right, directed by Lisa Cholodenko, Focus Features (2010).

Love Free Or Die, directed by Macky Alston, Reveal Productions (2012).

Making Love, directed by Arthur Hiller, IndieProd Company Productions (1982).

Orange Is the New Black, created by Jengi Kohan, Titled Productions (2013).

Prayers For Bobby, directed by Russell Mulcahy, Danile Sladek Entertainment (2009).

That Certain Summer, directed by Lamont Jackson, Universal Television (1972).

That's a Family, directed by Debra Chasnoff, Groundspark (2000).

Transparent, created by Jill Soloway, Amazon Studios (2013).

Trembling Before G-d , directed by Sandi Simcha Dubowski (2001).

Two Spirits, directed by Lydia Nibley, Say Yes Quickly Productions (2009).

Articles:

Advojonathan, "Pat Robertson Tells A Mother That Her Gay Son Is 'On Their Way To Hell.'" Glaad (2009) https://www.glaad.org/2009/06/16/pat-robertson-tells-a-mother-that-her-gay-son-is-on-their-way-to-hell

Bennett Smith, Meredith, "Carla Hale, Gay Teacher, Fired From Catholic High School After Being 'Outed' by Mother's Obituary." *Huffington Post* (2016). https://www.huffingtonpost.com/2013/04/18/carla-hale-gay-fired-teacher-catholic-high-school_n_3103853.html

Boyle, Mark, "North Carolina's transgender bathroom law may be repealed." *U.S.A. Today* (2016). https://www.usatoday.com/story/news/politics/2016/12/19/north-carolina-bathroom-bill/95615132/

Branch, John, "N.F.L. Prospect Michael Sam Proudly Says What Teammates Knew: He's Gay." *New York Times* (2014). https://www.nytimes.com/2014/02/10/sports/michael-sam-college-football-star-says-he-is-gay-ahead-of-nfl-draft.html

Brydum, Sunnivie, "Pope Francis Writes Private Letter To Gay Catholics." *TheAdvocate.com* (2013) https://www.advocate .com/politics/religion/2013/10/10/pope-francis-writes -private-letter-gay-catholics

Carey, Greg, "Rob Bell Comes Out For Marriage Equality." *Huffington Post* (2013) https://www.huffingtonpost.com/greg -carey/rob-bell-comes-gay-marriage_b_2898394.html

"Christianity and Homosexuality." Wikipedia. https://en.wikipedia .org/wiki/Christianity_and_homosexuality

El-Awady, Dr. Nadia, "Homosexuality in a Changing World: Are We Being Misinformed?" *IslamOnline.net* (2003). https: //archive.islamonline.net/?p=17507

Ejiofar, Clemente, "Gay Man Set Ablaze In Uganda Days After Anti Gay Bill Passed." *Naij.com* (2014). https://www.naija.ng /55056.html

"Federal Court Rules Employers Can't Fire People For Being Gay." *Lamda Legal* (2017). https://www.lambdalegal.org/blog /20170404_court-rules-employers-cant-discriminate-against -gay-employees

Fernandez, Manny, "School Officials Black Out Photo Of A Gay Student's Kiss." *New York Times* (2007). http://www.nytimes .com/2007/06/24/education/24yearbook.html

Hernandez, Greg, "Michael Buble Talks about his gay uncle and the lessons his parents taught him about gay people." *GregIn Hollywood.com* (2010). http://greginhollywood.com/michael -buble-talks-about-bullying-his-gay-uncle-and-the-lessons-his -parents-taught-him-about-gay-people-41298

"Homosexuality and Judiasm." Wikipedia. https://en.wikipedia .org/wiki/Homosexuality_and_Judaism

Hudson, David, "President Signs Executive Order To Protect LGBT workers." Whitehouse blog (2014), https://obamawhite house.archives.gov/blog/2014/07/21/president-obama -signs-new-executive-order-protect-lgbt-workers

Jaffe-Hoffman, Maaya, "For Transgender Teens, Jewish Rites of Passage Is Multilayered Transition." *Jewish News Syndicate* (2016). https://www.jns.org/for-transgender-teens-jewish-rite-of -passage-is-a-multi-layered-transition/

James Donaldson, Susan, " When Words Can Kill: 'That's So Gay.'" *ABCNEWS* (2009) http://abcnews.go.com/Health/MindMood News/story?id=7328091

Karlan, Sarah, "Gay High School Couple Wins 'Cutest Couple' For The Yearbook," *BuzzFeed* (2013). https://www.buzzfeed .com/skarlan/gay-high-school-couple-wins-cutest-couple-for -the-yearbook?utm_term=.sd6boVGAP#.jxNMA5xay

Lynch, Rene, "Put Gays and Lesbians Behind Electric Fence? Pastor's Sermon Goes Viral" *Los Angeles Times* (2012). http: //articles.latimes.com/2012/may/22/nation/la-na-nn-pastor -wants-to-put-gays-lesbians-behind-electrified-fence-20120522

Mai, Tram, "Pastor Calls For Killing Gays To End AIDS." *USA Today* (2014). https://www.usatoday.com/story/news/nation/2014 /12/04/pastor-calls-for-killing-gays-to-end-aids/19929973/

Malkin, Bonnie, "Gay Teenager Killed By Classmate in U.S." *The Telegraph* (2008). http://www.telegraph.co.uk/news/worldnews /1579834/Gay-teenager-killed-by-classmate-in-US.html

Margolin, Emma, "Kansas Lawmakers Retreat From Religious Liberty Bill." *MSNBC* (2014). http://www.msnbc.com/msnbc /kansas-gop-retreats-controversial-bill

Neuman, Scott, "Indiana's Governor Signs 'Religious Freedom' Bill." *NPR* (2015). https://www.npr.org/sections/thetwo-way

/2015/03/26/395583706/indianas-governor-signs-religious
-freedom-bill

Pilkington, Ed, "Tyler Clementi, Student Outed as Gay on
Internet, Jumps to His Death." *The Guardian* (2010). https://www
.theguardian.com/world/2010/sep/30/tyler-clementi
-gay-student-suicide

"Prop 8 Plaintiffs Kris Perry and Sandy Stier React To Ruling."
Kron 4 (2013). https://www.youtube.com/watch?v=0XVT
jR15bWQ

"Russia anti-gay Law: Putin sings bill banning 'propaganda of
nontraditional sexual relations.'" *The Associated Press* (2013).
https://www.thestar.com/news/world/2013/06/30/russia_
antigay_law_putin_signs_bill_banning_propaganda_of_non
-traditional_sexual_relations.html

Severson, Kim, "Backed By State Money, Georgia Scholarships
Go To Schools Banning Gays." *The New York Times* (2013).
http://www.nytimes.com/2013/01/21/education/geor
gia-backed-scholarships-benefit-schools-barring-gays.html

Shoichet, Catherine E and Halimah, Abdullah, "Arizona Gov.
Jan Brewer Vetoes Controversial Anti-gay Vill, SB 1062." *CNN*
.com (2014). https://www.cnn.com/2014/02/26/politics/arizo
na-brewer-bill/index.html

Wescott, Ben, "Australia Votes Yes To Same Sex Marriage."
CNN.com (2017). https://www.cnn.com/2017/11/14/asia/australia
-same-sex-marriage-yes/index.html

Acknowledgments

Thanks to my whole family for being supportive of my creative endeavors, including my sister Suzan Dougherty, who accidentally gave me the idea for the book. Also, to my late father, Nevzat, and my mom, Terry Karatas. My brothers, sisters, and in-laws (Sibel and Chris Gullo, Kenan and Michelle Karatas, and Kevin). All my aunts, uncles, and cousins here in the United States and in Turkey, and special thanks to Carlos Romani.

Thanks to all who helped make this book, a real passion project for me, a reality. To my awesome Literary agent Matt Wagner at Fresh Books Inc and to everyone at Skyhorse publishing: Nicole Frail, Emily Shields, Felicia Tsao.

Much of the material came from interviews and surveys I did, so thanks to all those who participated including: Maurie Davidson, Del and Caroline Shores, Bruce Vilanch, Liz Mullen, Debra Chasnoff, Davina Kotulski, Chely Wright, Tommy Starling, Wendy Montgomery Williams, Rick Foster, Kendall Evans, Connie Martinez, Robert Tejada, Dana Estrada, Rich Kosachiner, Adolfo Sotil, Frank Velasquez, Jason Stuart, *Lesléa Newman*, *Mike/Michelle*, Richard Vaughn and Tommy Woelfel,

Bill Poynter, Huck Walton, Jerrel Walls, Stuart Bell, Dr. Giella, Debra Coolhart, John Dennem, Reverend Dr. Sean B. Murray, Amy Shea, and Gary and Larry Lane.

Robin Marquis, who referred me to COLAGE, very special thanks to them, and other organizations like PFLAG, POP LUCK CLUB, and FAMILY EQUALITY COUNCIL.

Jana Ritter (who did some early editing for me) and Frank Hinterberger Steven Tyler, and Joseph Maake who did some proofreading for me.

A few others who have been helpful: Chuck Long, Jack Fitzgerald, Bill Poynter, Chris Gaida, Chuck Walter, Lorraine Epstein Marx, and Sheena O'Nair. There were so many more but the Orchestra is telling me to wrap it up. There is not enough space here to thank everyone who gave advice and helped me on this journey but please know it is appreciated.